The Ethics of Precision Medicine

NOTRE DAME STUDIES IN MEDICAL ETHICS
AND BIOETHICS

O. Carter Snead, series editor

DE NICOLA CENTER
for ETHICS AND CULTURE

The purpose of the Notre Dame Studies in Medical Ethics and Bioethics series, sponsored by the de Nicola Center for Ethics and Culture, is to publish works that explore the ethical, cultural, and public questions arising from advances in biomedical technology, the practice of medicine, and the biosciences.

THE ETHICS *of* PRECISION MEDICINE

The Problems of Prevention in Healthcare

PAUL SCHERZ

University of Notre Dame Press
Notre Dame, Indiana

Copyright © 2024 by the University of Notre Dame

Notre Dame, Indiana 46556

undpress.nd.edu

All Rights Reserved

Published in the United States of America

Library of Congress Control Number: 2024942067

ISBN: 978-0-268-20905-6 (Hardback)
ISBN: 978-0-268-20907-0 (WebPDF)
ISBN: 978-0-268-20908-7 (Epub3)

CONTENTS

| | *Preface* | vii |
| | *Acknowledgments* | xiii |

PART I
The Shift to Prevention

ONE	Suspicion of the Body	3
TWO	Sicken to Shun Sickness	13
THREE	Genetics and Risk	24
FOUR	Individuals and Populations	37
FIVE	Public Health Ethics and Clinical Ethics	45

PART II
Ethical Problems of Prevention

SIX	The Limitless Demand for Health	55
SEVEN	Managing Populations	63
EIGHT	The Obligation of Health	74
NINE	Exclusion and Elimination	82
TEN	Caring for the Statistical Other	87

PART III
Addressing the Problems of Prevention

ELEVEN	Prevention and the Social Determinants of Health	97
TWELVE	Regimen	106
THIRTEEN	Genomics in the Identification and Treatment of Disease	114
FOURTEEN	Institutions for Slow Medicine	124
	Notes	133
	Bibliography	163
	Index	191

PREFACE

Reducing health risk is the goal of much contemporary medical technology. For example, predicting risk is a prominent aim of the National Institutes of Health's (NIH) $1.5 billion, ten-year All of Us program. The program is enrolling one million people in a study that will sequence their genome and cross-reference it with their health records, biomarkers, and an ongoing analysis of diet and activity. Researchers hope that these data, when integrated, will give them a better sense of health risk factors. As Francis Collins, former head of the NIH, described, the agency seeks to gain "a considerably more useful estimate of your future risks of illness than is currently possible, enabling a personalized plan of preventive medicine to be established."[1] Participants in the All of Us program are the vanguard of a much larger movement to gain control of risk. Millions of people have sent their DNA samples to direct-to-consumer genome-sequencing companies like 23andMe. Among the many reasons they seek their DNA sequence is to predict their risks of chronic diseases. Many others track their health information with wearable devices, like Fitbits. These efforts exemplify what is called precision medicine, a research program that emerged after the Human Genome Project that attempts to target care to an individual's specific risk and disease characteristics.

Precision medicine, however, is merely the latest iteration of the much older framework of preventive medicine. For the last sixty years, medicine has sought to prevent disease or find diseases before they become apparent to the patient. Most people dutifully attend yearly checkups, receive blood tests for risk factors like cholesterol, and submit to cancer screening programs. Companies use gift cards or discounts on insurance to entice their workers to enroll in wellness programs. Managing risk is already a central aim of medicine, and its role in healthcare is only set to grow, shifting the traditional goals of clinical medicine away from treating individual illness. Now medicine is treating population risk. As Francis Collins's words indicate, precision medicine is just the next step in preventive medicine, seeking risk not only in physiology but in the genome.

The value of prevention seems obvious: by catching diseases early, medicine should have an easier time curing them. There are clearly scenarios in which surveillance yields large benefits, such as treatment of high blood pressure, or mammography for women with a familial history of breast cancer. As the number of conditions surveilled and treated expands, however, problems emerge. More and more people find themselves at risk, caught between health and disease. They are not ill but have the anxiety of illness. Though having no symptoms, they take pharmaceuticals, undergo prophylactic surgeries, or are otherwise medically managed. These interventions themselves are not without their own dangers: side effects from pharmaceuticals; complications of surgeries; and the health effects of anxieties. An increasing number of voices within medicine are challenging the preventive framework because the effectiveness of our current preventive strategies is unclear, with clinical trials showing that many risk-reducing pharmaceuticals and screenings may have little if any impact on patients' overall survival. There are also social dangers, such as the expense of additional surgeries and pharmaceuticals straining an already overburdened health system. Moreover, managing population risks requires increased surveillance of both doctors and patients, leading to new forms of social control. While certain targeted forms of risk reduction have undeniable medical value, as chapter 13 will discuss, expanding this paradigm in such a way that it seeks to control any and all risk creates dangers. Society ends up facing a rash of overtreatment, overdiagnosis, and social control.

These concerns cannot be dismissed as antiscience or antimedicine. The analysis in this book follows the lead of mainstream medical journals in their concerns over prevention leading to overdiagnosis and overtreatment, such as the *BMJ*'s "Too Much Medicine" initiative and *JAMA Internal Medicine*'s "Less Is More" series. Moreover, respected organizations like the Cochrane Collaboration and the U.S. Preventive Services Task Force, which are among the most reliable data analysts in medicine, publish meta-analyses casting doubt on the benefits of many preventive interventions. The debate is not over science as such but over undecided questions within science, which raise broader ethical questions surrounding what values lead us to accept the consequences and risks of over- or undertreatment. The question driving this book is why, with so much controversy surrounding particular medicines and guidelines, the goal of prevention has been taken for granted by policymakers, patients, and ethicists. The taken-for-granted nature of these efforts in the face of conflicting evidence indicates that the paradigm of prevention aligns with ethical and social values that need to be explored and questioned in more depth.

While a growing number of books and articles by physicians, medical historians, and critical theorists explore the problems of current paradigms of preventive and precision medicine, there has yet to be an ethical analysis of these phenomena. That is the goal of this book: to examine the ethics of precision medicine in relation to the broader framework of preventive healthcare. It does so through the lens of virtue ethics.[2] The goal of virtue ethics is to help people live a flourishing life, in which flourishing includes physical, social, intellectual, and spiritual components. Virtue ethics has been a resource for many religious and philosophical traditions, each of which has distinct pictures of exactly what that flourishing, fulfilled life will look like.[3] All agree, though, that flourishing requires not just particular right actions but also the development of certain character traits and emotional dispositions. A person cannot flourish if constantly overwhelmed by fear or anger or consistently battling temptations to steal or break commitments to others. The individual has to become the type of person who genuinely enjoys doing the good actions that lead to individual and communal flourishing. These character traits that are part of a flourishing life are called virtues. There are many, but classical virtue ethics focused on four major or cardinal virtues: Justice is the desire to give everyone their due. Temperance ensures that one has healthy, reasonable appetites in relation to physical pleasures like food, alcohol, or sex. Courage allows one to control fear of danger. Overseeing all of these other virtues is prudence, or practical wisdom, which integrates these other traits in order to determine and execute a good action in a particular situation.

In the specific context of medicine, virtue ethics has examined the dispositions necessary for the medical practitioner and patient to jointly respond to the suffering caused by illness.[4] These are the virtues that help the patient rightly relate to his body and suffering, and hopefully ultimately lead to healing. The medical practitioner must be just in order to fulfill her duties to the patient and society. Training shapes the practitioner to undergo the hardships of long hours, forming temperance. A practitioner must have courage in the face of patients' potential death. Integrating these traits is clinical judgment, which serves as a medical version of prudence.

I argue that preventive medicine, when poorly done, can harm individual and communal flourishing. The book traces three dangers to flourishing. First, the anxiety of risk as patients are defined as ill before they exhibit any symptoms affects their relationship to their bodies, causing fears that undermine courage and the peaceful enjoyment of the present. Second, traditional understandings of the relationship between doctor and patient are undermined as medicine focuses on managing population risk, undermining justice and its associated virtues like solidarity. Third, the demand for medical intervention to shape population risk affects politics and the power structures within medicine, as institutions are forced into ever-greater attempts at surveillance and control of both practitioners and patients. These new institutional commitments undermine the practitioner's prudence. Risk-based prevention might serve many individuals poorly and can lead to the exclusion of those most at risk.

My criticism seeks to serve a constructive aim: to ensure that the advanced technologies of precision medicine are used well in ways that support human flourishing. Not all strategies of prevention raise these problems. I distinguish between two paradigms of prevention. The first might be called the medical management of population risk. This is the form discussed in the first paragraph: it scans individuals for risk factors or early disease and attempts to treat them before they become worse. The second approach to prevention might be called the remediation of unhealthy structures. This would involve changing aspects of social and personal life that we know predispose people to disease, such as poverty. The latter paradigm is frequently tied to the idea of the social determinants of health. As the last part of the book will discuss, I support this mode of prevention, although I eschew the language of social determinants, because the word *social* is closely tied in policy documents to the idea of managing populations through medical efforts. Truly addressing social risks requires shifting social structures as well as how individuals structure their own lives and habits. The book emphasizes developing structures that help people to embody the virtues of justice, solidarity, and temperance. Crucially, medicine as a discipline has relatively little to say about how to justly organize society or what leads to a flourishing life. Risk management is useful in many situations, but we must develop the prudence and institutions that will allow us to use it well.

On a final note, the book will largely discuss noninfectious diseases, as these have been the drivers of postwar preventive efforts and contemporary precision medicine. Infectious disease prevention raises different questions concerning the common good and individual action. Very little will be said about things like common childhood vaccinations, of which I am a proponent, because they are not as tied into the efforts to control noninfectious diseases. I will discuss recent experiences with Covid-19, however, insofar as the public health response to Covid illuminates more general issues in regard to prevention.

The book has three parts that follow the preface. The introductory chapter explores the concept of health and how medicine traditionally responded to the disruption of health, before describing why preventive medicine itself disrupts the experience of health in damaging ways. Chapters 2 through 5 trace the historical reasons for the shift to prevention and its current instantiation in precision medicine, through the lenses of medical research, genetics, and medical ethics. These chapters will introduce pragmatic problems created by prevention and its statistical vision of the person, giving an overview of contemporary disputes in the broader literature. Chapters 6 through 10, the heart of the ethical analysis, will delve into the conceptual and ethical problems of preventive medicine. The goal of reducing risk has no inherent rational limit, and thus interventions tend to continuously expand, undermining the prudence seen in approaches to health that respond to disease while still accepting human finitude. Reducing risk requires an increasing demand for control of potential patients, leading to a changed understanding of justice. The last four chapters develop a more positive picture of prevention by describing movements that address structural risks to health as well as productive uses of risk analysis in healthcare. These chapters point the way to a more reasonable approach to prevention that safeguards human flourishing.

ACKNOWLEDGMENTS

Many people contributed to the completion of this work. My thanks go to the School of Theology and Religious Studies at the Catholic University of America, which provided a fertile ground for conversations and allowed me to take leaves to write parts of this book. I owe special thanks to Jeanatan Hall, a graduate research assistant who edited many of the chapters. Events at the Institute for Advanced Studies in Culture at the University of Virginia, where I was a Visiting Faculty Fellow while I wrote this book, have fostered many of the theoretical developments in the book, especially through conversations with Joseph Davis, Justin Mutter, Matthew Crawford, William Hasselberger, Mark Hoipkemeier, and Tal Brewer.

I would also like to thank Jesse Couenhoven, Gerald McKenny, and Neil Arner for their invitation to participate in a grant project and a writing group, as well as the John Templeton Foundation, who, through grant #61661, made this work possible. Christiana Zenner also took part in that writing group, which gave invaluable feedback on much of the book. As part of the grant, Ted Porter served as an adviser on the historical portions of the book and Nortin Hadler advised me on many of the more technical discussions of preventive medicine. Their guidance enriched those sections.

Work on this manuscript was also partially supported by my participation in activities funded by a grant from the McDonald Agape Foundation (Grant title: Out of Our Meds? Building a Theological and Moral Framework for the Use of Medications). Through the grant's events, I received comments on the project from Farr Curlin, Warren Kinghorn, Kavin Rowe, Mary Hirschfeld, Bradley Gregory, Brett McCarty, Stanley Hauerwas, Peter MacDonald, Macarius Donneyong, Dima Qato, and Michael Pencina.

These conversations were crucial for developing my discussions regarding the Covid pandemic and the influence of risk on the healing relationship.

Parts of the book were presented at the University of Virginia's Department of Religious Studies and its Center for Health Humanities and Ethics; the Instituto de Estudos Politicos at Universidade Catolica Portuguesa; the Grefenstette Center for Ethics in Science, Technology and Law at Duquesne University; Santa Clara University; a webinar for the McGrath Institute for Church Life at the University of Notre Dame; the University of St. Thomas; Franciscan Missionaries of Our Lady University; the Lumen Christi Institute at the University of Chicago; the Conference on Medicine and Religion; the Catholic Health Association's Theology and Ethics Colloquium; the Society of Christian Ethics; the Center for Bioethics and Human Dignity at Trinity International University; and the American Academy of Religion. I am grateful to these organizations for these opportunities to write the relevant sections as well as valuable feedback I received through discussions at these presentations.

Christian Bioethics and Oxford University Press have graciously given me permission to use sections of "Risk, Health, and Physical Enhancement: The Dangers of Health Care as Risk Reduction for Christian Bioethics," *Christian Bioethics* 26, no. 2 (2020): 145–62, throughout the book as well as ideas and some paragraphs from "No Acceptable Losses: Risk, Prevention, and Justice," *Christian Bioethics* 29, no. 2 (2023): 164–75, copyright 2020 and 2023, published by Oxford University Press, on behalf of The Journal of Christian Bioethics, Inc., all rights reserved. I would also like to thank Emily King, three anonymous reviewers, and the staff at the University of Notre Dame Press for their suggestions and other help in bringing this publication to completion.

Finally, I thank my family for the support they have given me through this project, both in giving me the time it takes to write and in being there when I could no longer bear to look at another word. My mother, Elizabeth Scherz, has been an amazing support to our family life. My wife, China, and my children, Iggy and Lucy, have been incredibly patient as I continually point out aspects of risk in our daily life.

Part I

The Shift to Prevention

ONE

Suspicion of the Body

Emerging technologies provide startling possibilities for detecting health risks. Take, for example, the surveillance capacities used in a study by the Pioneer 100 Wellness Project.[1] These researchers gathered an incredible amount of data from 108 participants: researchers sequenced participants' genomes; sampled the bacteria in their gut; tested their blood for 643 metabolites and 262 proteins every three months; and asked them to wear a Fitbit to track activity and sleep. They combined and analyzed these data in light of the latest research in genetics and medicine.

What did the researchers and participants discover when monitored in such detail? They found that no one is healthy. Almost everyone in the study was at risk for something: half were prediabetic, almost no one got enough vitamin D, eighty-one had high mercury levels, and one had a possible problem with iron metabolism. One participant, a health-conscious venture capitalist who ran triathlons and already devoted a lot of time to wellness, was surprised to learn he was prediabetic. It was not that the subjects had undiscovered diseases; relatively few active diseases appeared. Instead, participants had undiscovered risks for disease. Their health disappeared into risk.

All was not lost for the participants, though. The investigators offered to address such risks through intensive coaching, a model they turned into a now-defunct start-up company providing monitoring and coaching for (initially) only $3,499 a year. These coaches suggested interventions to manage the risks detected in the analysis, like supplements, medications, and even medical procedures. Through ongoing action and an increased regimentation of their life, participants' hidden risks could be managed and controlled.

While this project involved only a few people, it embodies a broader paradigm called precision medicine, which seeks to use genetics and other advanced technologies to identify health risks. Precision medicine is set to become more entrenched in science and medicine as governments complete massive projects such as the National Institutes of Health's All of Us study or the U.K.'s Biobank project. These projects seek much more knowledge of the risk factors embedded in our genomes than we currently have. This precision medicine will combine knowledge of genetics, physiology, and lifestyle to prevent disease.

Yet the sheer prevalence of risk in the Pioneer 100 Wellness Project research cohort should give us pause in our project to replace health with risk. How do we live and engage healthcare when no one is healthy? Given that the Pioneer 100 and All of Us projects are only manifestations of a broader paradigm of prevention, what is the relationship between prevention, risk, and health? This first chapter will begin to explore some of these issues, starting with a phenomenological definition of health that will guide the discussion in the rest of the book. This definition reveals how medicine based in prevention challenges our naïve conception of health, as well as the dangers that lie in efforts to predict and address health risks before they arise.

Health as Absence of Disease

Traditionally, medicine aimed at health, seeking primarily to make sick people healthy again.[2] Health, however, is a difficult concept to define, because a person does not have a distinct experience of health.[3] Health is an absence: it is an absence of negative bodily experiences, since when a person is healthy, there are no dissonances or pains that draw his attention. Health is "a state of unawareness where the subject and his body are one."[4] Because of this inattention, "our enjoyment of good health is constantly concealed from us."[5] Ancient doctors spoke of health as a harmony, or balance.[6] Usually, they drew on theories of the balance of the humors, but these theories involve the same sense of nothing being noticeably out of order. Fredrik Svenaeus has called it a feeling of being at home in the body, meaning that we do not feel out of place in our body.[7] Even more reductionist, medical understandings of disease define health in contrast to dysfunction or an abnormal range of values. In all of these understandings, disease is the primary experience. Health is merely disease's absence.

Pain or the failure of the body draws one's attention.[8] Otherwise, the body freely manifests a person's action into the world, seemingly transparent to the person's will. The body is one's tool for engaging the world, as Aristotle suggests in describing it as an organic body, a body made of tools.[9] Describing the body as a tool does not instrumentalize it but instead recalls the experience of the craftsman whose commonly used tools become almost an extension of the self; or the blind person's cane; or the short-sighted person's glasses.[10] These tools are absorbed into the experience of the body and ultimately disappear from awareness. The craftsman notices his tools only when they break or malfunction.[11] They cease to be a transparent medium of his action into the world and are brought to his attention as a problem, or something that he needs to address. It is the same with the body; a person attends to it when it ceases to function or brings pain to her attention, while its erasure from attention is a characteristic of health.[12] The focal attention on pain, dysfunction, or limitation is the experience of disease. In disease, the body becomes other to one's will.[13]

Even an experience of pain or discomfort does not necessarily mean that disease is present or that the person feels the need to seek medical care, or even that she should be concerned. There are defined rhythms to health, quirks of a season or of a period in life; to continue the tool metaphor, a car might take longer to start in the winter or a lock might need a jiggle when you turn the key without these being indications of a broken car or lock.[14] As I write this section, my nose is running due to allergies, which always appear in the spring as flowers bloom. The discomfort of a runny nose or a sinus headache is not strange or unpredictable. I am not concerned by these symptoms, as they are how my body usually responds to the cycle of seasons. Similarly, I do not grow concerned over a minor cold in the midst of winter, as I expect to get a cold at some time during these months. Women are especially familiar with this rhythmic nature of healthy bodily processes, with predictable changes occurring over both the short term (monthly cycles) and over life as a whole (puberty, pregnancy, menopause). Even serious discomfort does not inspire concern if the cause is apparent. If I drink too much and am laid up much of the next morning, I do not blame my body, but my foolish choices. The discomfort is a natural response to my actions. If I eat at a dodgy restaurant and spend the next day with stomach pain, my feeling of my body as predictable and reliable is not necessarily disrupted, and I seek medical care only if the stomach pain lasts longer than usual. These kinds of expected, rhythmic discomforts do not lead to medical care. Instead, people turn to nonmedical remedies, like sleep, chicken soup, the BRAT diet, Neti pots, a hot toddy, and so forth; or they turn to the common over-the-counter pharmacopeia for support: aspirin, Sudafed, Nyquil.[15]

Similarly, not all limitations are a disease or indicate the absence of health. If I am out of breath after hiking up a hill that I used to climb with ease, I recognize that I am out of shape, not unhealthy. I will just need to exercise more if I want to climb it without difficulty. As people age, they face more and more limitations and aches in the body. This can be accepted as part of the rhythmic nature of health, with a rhythm extending over the whole life course.[16] There are some limitations to physical endurance and performance that appear no matter what one's physical fitness or health; humans only run so fast for so long or stay up for so many continuous nights in a row. These are accepted as limitations of the body, as what one expects of it, unless one seeks to exceed the human condition.[17]

Even states that most people would see as requiring medical care, like disability or chronic disease, can still lead to an equilibrium recognized as a new form of health.[18] Many people with disabilities do not even recognize them as a source of limitations but merely as a different way of being in a body.[19] Even those with chronic illness can reach normal states of comfortable action in the world once they are medically stabilized. They accept their new bodily equilibria as their state of health.

The experience of illness or disease emerges only when the body ceases to be a predictable medium for acting in the world. In such situations, severe pain and limitation disorient the person. The world and the body become alien, other to the self. The person no longer feels at home in the world. This disorientation causes fear and distress, and, if intense enough, it leads to suffering. It is this moment of suffering that sets the stage for the clinical encounter. Experiences of unexpected limitation, or pain with which they cannot cope, drive the person to seek medical help and to become a patient.[20] In the face of disease, the medical practitioner steps forward and professes to be able and willing to help the person address her bodily suffering.[21] The practice of medicine addresses suffering by seeking to restore health. If not capable of restoring the full function experienced before illness, it at least tries to banish as much of the alienating nature of disease as possible, to reorient the patient to her body. It does this by explaining the causes of the patient's condition, removing confusion; or it predicts the course of disease, removing uncertainty; or it reduces pain, restores function, and seeks to help the patient recognize her new equilibrium of health so that she can return to feeling at home in the body. In accounts of medical ethics dependent on virtue, it is this commitment to seek the patient's good by overcoming suffering that drives the need and creates the structure for medical virtues.[22]

The Body and Prevention

So far, I have analyzed a number of ways that the body may come to focal awareness: major illness, disability, seasonal complaints, or changes over the life course. All of these can be reasons to engage medicine. There is of course the trip to the ER due to severe chest pain, but also advice on addressing allergies, or physical therapy to minimize the aches of the aging body. In all of these cases, the patient's relationship to his body is disrupted, leading him to seek medical care.

This book addresses none of these cases, except only incidentally. If, as you read it, you think of counterexamples to my arguments that arise from disability or disease, please remember that I am explicitly ruling out those experiences from consideration.[23] This book instead highlights a relatively recent way that the body becomes other. In this new approach, medicine takes someone who otherwise would feel in good health, at home in his body, and causes him to see it as potentially dangerous. This is the experience of medical prevention.[24]

The goal of preventive medicine, as well as its latest incarnation, precision medicine, is to ward off future illness by finding it in its early stages or finding precursors to its full manifestation in the present when it can, in theory, be easily treated. Patients are promised that they can prevent the disruption of their health, the loss of the quality of feeling at home in their body, and even the loss of their life through early action. Generally this early action occurs through a regime of testing and analysis of the body. The body is objectified in order to find early signs of dysfunction. For example, men might have a PSA test to detect early stages of prostate cancer. Women get mammograms to catch breast cancer early. People examine moles and other skin blemishes to ferret out potential melanoma. Blood pressure predicts future cardiovascular disease. And many people pay attention to weight to try to wrestle their Body Mass Index (BMI) out of the range of risk for diabetes, heart disease, and other ailments. Much of medical practice is now aimed at detecting risks or emergent diseases.[25]

Oddly, in trying to prevent disease, the patient is thrown into a state very similar to the experience of disease. Say one gets a PSA test or mammogram. While some might give it no thought, many other patients are assailed by anxiety as they await the results, wondering if their body hides a tumor.[26] This anxiety is deepened for the many people who will receive a positive result that calls for a biopsy. They will become even more concerned as they wait for the result of their surgical procedure. Even if it is a false positive and the patients return to their daily lives, they have been plunged into the experience of illness. The body became alienated, a source of risk.

Other forms of detecting risk share this quality of distancing the person from the body. Examining moles, checking weight, taking blood pressure, all make the body into an object for analysis. The body ceases to be the tool used without thought and becomes an object of focal awareness. Many of these techniques for objectifying the body do so by quantifying aspects of it, turning health into a composite of BMI, blood pressure, blood sugar, and other scores. Public health campaigns and workplace wellness programs encourage us to know our numbers, seeing an important truth about health in those biostatistics. No longer is the absence of distress or discomfort enough to indicate health: experience must match the objective facts. In many cases, this sets up a conflict with an unruly body as, for example, a person's weight or blood pressure refuses to drop no matter what he tries or his numbers rise back into the danger zone as soon as he hits a stressful patch.

This form of medicine sets up a relationship to the body that can only be characterized as suspicion, the fear of the dangers the body might hide despite its seeming health. Many patients, upon receiving results indicating disease or predisease, cease to trust their body.[27] This suspicion is perhaps best exemplified in the Quantified Self (QS) movement.[28] Members of this movement seek self-knowledge through quantification, a goal that is facilitated by the development of new health-monitoring devices like the Fitbit. Wearable tracking devices allow individuals to monitor huge amounts of health data: pulse, blood pressure, sleep rhythms, calories burned, number of steps taken, and so on. QS enthusiasts fear that felt experience and phenomenological analysis are illusory; truth can come only through the objectification and mathematical analysis of aspects of the self, especially the body. I fear that such a framework can only become disempowering and alienating. Even if one possesses one's own numerical readouts, this is no true self-knowledge. As coming chapters will show, this quantitative knowledge must be interpreted through a contested domain of expert knowledge. To know one's risk, one must ignore one's subjective understanding of one's health and defer, not even to the expert judgment of the doctor, but to complex statistical manipulations of large datasets emerging from epidemiological studies and clinical trials that even most medical professionals are not competent to understand, let alone judge.[29]

It is important to distinguish this entry of otherwise healthy people into an experience of health risk similar to a state of disease from another experience of risk that arises out of our relational nature. Because we arise out of a family and are descended from others, the diseases of relatives can feel like our own. Having a father die of an early heart attack can alienate a man from his body. Seeing a mother or a cousin struggle with breast cancer can lead a woman to suspicion of her own breasts. In these ways, medicine does not intervene to drive an experience of risk. The loss of those close to us always disrupts our world, and this disruption becomes even worse when they die of diseases recognized as hereditary. Later chapters will discuss how genetics and screening technologies may fruitfully address this disruption. In such cases, medicine and screening step in to address alienation in a way different from the broader influence of risk-based prevention that I discuss here.[30]

Medical prevention, in contrast, leads into an odd territory in which we recapitulate the phenomenological experience of illness in order to prevent entering into that experience of illness in the future. It prevents in the sense of warding off future disease. Yet the word *prevent* in early modern

English contained an ambiguity, like many other important medical terms, such as the *pharmakon* that means both medicine and poison. This other sense of *prevent* that precision medicine also fulfills means "to hasten, bring about, or put before the time or prematurely; to anticipate," or "to act as if (the event or time) had already come."[31] This is an older, now obsolete definition of *prevent*, but one often found in the King James Bible. For example, "Mine eyes *prevent* the night watches, that I might meditate in thy word."[32] Or compare the Douay-Rheims translation of Esther 8:10: "And these letters which were sent in the king's name, were sealed with his ring, and sent by posts: who were to run through all the provinces, to *prevent* the former letters with new messages." In both passages, *prevent* means to anticipate or to move faster than.

Prevent comes from the Latin *praevenire*, a word that combines "to come" and "before." It points to a relationship to a future occurrence. People can relate to this future in two ways: either by anticipating it or by rejecting it. Though seemingly opposite, these divergent responses can oddly coalesce: risk-based medical prevention acts as if illness has already arrived, prematurely creating the phenomenal experience of illness before the state of the body drives one into it, and thus anticipating it. The patient submits to the pain and inconveniences of treatment before forced to by the pains of illness; it is done, though, in an attempt to reject future illness. The preventive patient is disoriented, alienated from the body before suffering occurs. Honestly confronting the alienating quality of illness when we are struck by disease does not raise many ethical or philosophical problems. It seems dangerous, though, to set up this suspicious alterity as an all-encompassing and ongoing framework for relating to the body and health.

The Gnostic Body

Recognizing the body as other is not alien to the Western understanding of the body, especially as interpreted in light of the Christian tradition. For example, in Paul's writings, sinful desires can make the body seem other, just as much as the experience of disease: "I see in my members another law at war with the law of my mind, making me captive to the law of sin that dwells in my members. Wretched man that I am! Who will rescue me from this body of death?"[33] In most of Christian history, the alienated body became the basis for the charitable response of medical care or the penitential response of asceticism. In the case of disease, the Christian attempts to heal the body, thus relieving suffering and restoring balance. In the case of sinful desires, the Christian tries to bring the passions into alignment with reason through exercises directed toward temperance.[34] Both of these strategies aim at reintegrating the self, allowing the body or the passions to disappear from the focal awareness of them caused by alienation. Even if these efforts fail at reintegrating the self in the moment, the Pauline vision aims at an ultimate reconciliation in which this same mortal flesh is transformed into a spiritual body where the alienation between body and spirit can never again occur: "For while we are still in this tent, we groan under our burden, because we wish not to be unclothed but to be further clothed, so that what is mortal may be swallowed up by life."[35] The body ultimately will be valued for itself and its contribution to the fullness of the person.

There is another approach to this alterity, however, one that parodies the Pauline vision. This is the Gnostic approach that denies the ultimate value of the body, that denies the possibility of reintegrating the body and psyche because the body is seen as ultimately alien to the self.[36] Gnosticism was a movement of diverse groups in the first centuries after Christ. Generally, Gnostic groups rejected this world, viewing it as a material realm in which the soul or spirit was trapped, and thus rejected the physical body itself as the most immanent manifestation of this material prison. The material world was not their true home. Gnostic knowledge or rites promised a spiritual escape from the body into a realm beyond the cosmos. In the contemporary world, transhumanism is frequently compared to Gnosticism in that it promises to use technology to escape the limitations of the errant body.[37] The transhumanist body will not become reintegrated with spirit, as in the Pauline vision, but will become completely subservient to the individual's autonomous will to the point of complete replacement by technology.

Precision and preventive medicine threatens to embody the Gnostic framework of suspicion of the body in a form different from transhumanism, although still technologically mediated. The body is again experienced as other, something that is dangerous, something always to treat with suspicion. The person is not at home in the body. To confront this alterity, the body must be watched. Medicine must place the body under continuous surveillance through blood pressure cuffs, Fitbits, scales, mammograms, colonoscopies, stool DNA tests, or PSA tests to find true knowledge. Once the truth of the body is seen in a verified risk, interventions like surgeries or risk-reducing medications are applied to eliminate that risk. The body is a danger that must be controlled by medical technologies. Unfortunately, precision medicine offers no salvation from this experience of alienation; unlike transhumanism or ancient Gnosticism, there is no escape from this alterity through technological means or spiritual enlightenment. The body will always be at risk.[38] Discovery and treatment of risk just mean that one continues to be at risk, usually a higher risk.[39] Even if no risk is found in a test, the patient still must return in one, two, or five years to repeat the test. There is an unending demand for surveillance and control, which, in turn, leads to continuing experiences of fear and alienation.

— The next three chapters will describe the developments that led to the current preoccupation with medical risk, discussing how we arrived at our current situation of a suspicion of the body. A first reason, examined in the second chapter, is the development of a focus on risk factors and mass screening programs that attempt to find and address disease before it strikes. The third chapter will then examine the new obsession with the deepest risks of all, those associated with our genome. The Human Genome Project promised to reveal the truth of our bodies, the "Book of Life," and it has found that this truth is one of risk, or so it claims.[40] These chapters will each focus on one troubling aspect of the preventive approach. Chapter 2 will examine how disease is brought into the present through the side effects of risk reduction. Chapters 3 and 4, addressing the statistical vision of the body that emerges from medical and genetic descriptions of risk, will also explain the disappearance of the lived body from an understanding of illness. One's own body is understood as an instance of the metrics of the population, so that the body disappears into statistics. One cannot feel at home on a normal curve. These overviews of recent historical investigations prepare the ground for the later discussion of ethical problems in precision medicine.

TWO

Sicken to Shun Sickness

Like as, to make our appetites more keen,
With eager compounds we our palate urge;
As, to prevent our maladies unseen,
We sicken to shun sickness when we purge;
Even so, being full of your ne'er-cloying sweetness,
To bitter sauces did I frame my feeding;
And sick of welfare found a kind of meetness
To be diseas'd, ere that there was true needing.
—William Shakespeare, "Sonnet 118"

    The most common interaction a person has with medicine is the yearly checkup. If a patient does not have a chronic disease, then most of the appointment will be taken up with discussing different physiological numbers or tests: reviewing blood pressure, cholesterol, weight, bone density, mammograms, or colonoscopies. These discussions aim at prevention. Little if any time in the appointment is spent in addressing actual physical complaints, because if a patient were actually ill she would have made a special appointment or gone to one of the cheaper clinics attached to pharmacies. The clinical encounter for many people revolves around analyzing risks.

    This framework for the clinical encounter is relatively recent, arising within the last century. Prior generations of patients sought out doctors only when they were ill.[1] Of course, prior generations of doctors could not provide much that would prevent future illness (and little enough to cure actually existing ailments), but they were not expected to. This chapter will examine this shift in medical care toward prevention, focusing on two of the major disease classes driving the rise of preventive medicine: cardiovascular disease and cancer. After this brief historical overview, the chapter will outline some of the problems with this paradigm of medicine, including its generation of new kinds of risk. Emphasizing prevention threatens to alienate one from the body, as the last chapter discussed, but the dangers of anticipating illness are not limited to the psychological realm. Efforts at prevention always run the risk of themselves bringing about physiological illness. Risk-reducing medicines have side effects, and prophylactic surgeries threaten complications. Even screening tests bear their own dangers, like radiation from mammography or overdiagnosis due to false positives. Many doctors are now asking whether the medical benefits of some of these preventive exercises outweigh their risks. Addressing this question will require examining the role of thinking in terms of populations in this paradigm of medicine, and the conundrums that population-based thinking creates for individual patients.

Cardiovascular Disease and Risk

By the middle of the twentieth century, infectious diseases were no longer leading causes of death because of better nutrition, increased sanitation, and the introduction of vaccines and antibiotics.[2] Instead, noninfectious diseases, like cancer or diabetes, occupied medical attention, as they still do today. Chief among these noninfectious diseases was heart disease. In 1900, pneumonia, tuberculosis, and diarrhea all came before heart disease in the ranks of causes of death, but by the 1920s heart disease was consistently the leading cause of death.[3] By midcentury, heart disease accounted for double the number of deaths of the next highest killer and still leads today, although cancer is catching up.[4] More troublingly to people in the mid-twentieth century, cardiovascular disease did not primarily kill the marginalized, as had many infectious diseases. Instead, heart attacks could strike down the most powerful men in society in their prime. There was, and remains in some quarters, a stereotype suggesting that more powerful men, like CEOs, were especially vulnerable to heart attacks because of the stress of their jobs.[5] Medical research therefore expended its efforts not only on treating cardiovascular disease but also on preventing it in the first place. Three aspects of this research drove the development of preventive medicine: the idea of disease as hidden in the healthy body, the concept of risk factors, and corporate profitability.

First, there was a reconceptualization of heart disease as an entity that exists in nascent form even in healthy bodies. A landmark study of Korean War casualties brought this hidden danger to light.[6] The researchers performed autopsies on soldiers who had died in combat, finding that many of the bodies were already showing signs of atherosclerosis, the hardening of the arteries that can lead to many cardiovascular problems. These were mostly soldiers in their early twenties, whereas heart disease did not strike until at least middle age. Long before any medical problems emerged, the disease was already developing. The researchers became suspicious of the body that did not reveal its truth through felt symptoms.

A second central moment in this story of preventive medicine is the Framingham Heart Study, a long-term longitudinal study that followed 4,494 adults in the town of Framingham, Massachusetts, through a set of health exams.[7] The study's long duration and large scale allowed investigators to examine characteristics correlated to disease that might not be apparent in a short-term, small-scale study. Because of its length, researchers discovered which characteristics and behaviors existing at the beginning of the study would be correlated with the emergence of disease later in the study. Its size allowed them to notice characteristics and behaviors whose correlation might emerge only through statistical analysis. They sought physiological signs or behaviors that did not always directly lead to disease, perhaps doing so only a slight percentage of the time, but still seemed to contribute to it. They called these signs, like high cholesterol, elevated blood pressure, or smoking, risk factors. These risk factors do not deterministically cause illness; we all know of people like my grandmother who smoked, cooked with bacon fat, and subsisted seemingly largely on jelly beans for her last fifteen years, yet lived with little illness or mental impairment until she rapidly declined after a fall at age ninety-two. There are always people who will lie on the lucky tail of the statistical curve. Still, these factors raise the risk of bad outcomes. Such risk factors were hidden from casual observation, emerging only when examined at the level of the population through statistical techniques. In other words, individual risk emerges only when the patient is seen in light of a population. Over the course of the twentieth century, these risk factors themselves became indistinguishable from disease in medical practice and are now frequently called prediseases, like prediabetes, or have themselves been defined as diseases, like mild hypertension. These diseases can be seen only at the level of the population.[8]

A third factor in the turn to risk reduction is the pharmaceutical industry. Indeed, some commentators view pharmaceutical companies as perhaps the most important driver in the turn to the treatment of risk.[9] Some of today's most popular drug classes are those that do not so much treat disease as treat risks, such as blood pressure or cholesterol levels. Pharmaceutical companies have long supported research into risk factors and have driven medicine's focus on risk factors. For example, once Merck, Sharpe, and Dohme developed Diuril, an effective drug for lowering blood pressure, in the 1950s, they started marketing campaigns in concert with patient advocacy and expert groups to call for the treatment of moderate hypertension.[10] Diuril and its manufacturer's publicity were central to the increased focus on hypertension. In contrast, if there was no effective pharmaceutical agent that addressed a risk factor, that risk factor was often ignored. Hence, even though the Framingham Study showed that cholesterol levels were risk factors for heart disease, it was not until the development of the first statin that they became a target for preventive medicine.[11]

The shift to a focus on risk was a conscious strategy on the part of the pharmaceutical industry. As Pfizer's chief of operations said in 1957 in response to the success of curative treatments like antibiotics: "There seems to be an important lesson here for the drug industry. . . . As the industry does a good job of producing efficacious drugs and helps to win a given campaign . . . the net result is to limit the potential market."[12] If a disease is cured, patients no longer need medication for it, thereby foreclosing continued sales. In contrast, once people are at risk for a disease, they remain at risk. Therefore, they will need to keep taking medications for the rest of their lives. Drugs targeting risk, unlike drugs that cure, do not eliminate their markets. Further, these drugs treat, not only those with a disease or who will certainly get a disease, but also all those who would never get the disease. The category of those at risk for a disease is always larger than the category of those who have a disease unless the risk is 100 percent, in which case we usually do not term it a risk but a certain cause. Indeed, clinical trials for risk reduction, which are predominantly funded and run by pharmaceutical companies, are designed to ensure that as many people as possible qualify for treatment.[13] For all of these reasons, a focus on risk reduction has led to an increase in prescriptions. Thus cardiovascular risk became a target because of a suspicion of the body driven in part by the discovery of statistically derived risk factors and in part through the interests of the pharmaceutical industry.

Cancer Screening

Another paradigm for risk reduction is cancer screening. Just as cardiovascular disease grew in prominence in line with a falling infectious disease burden, so did cancer. As more people lived longer, more people died of cancer, making it the second leading cause of death by midcentury. It has nearly overtaken heart disease in recent years.[14] Already by the end of the nineteenth and the early twentieth centuries, doctors focused on catching cancer as early as possible and then engaging in radical treatment.[15] This strategy drew on a developmental model of cancer. This theory postulated, with little epidemiological evidence, that all cancers follow relatively the same disease course. They start as abnormal cells, then become larger tumors, then result in aggressive metastatic disease spreading through the body. The key idea was that cancers all become more dangerous and harder to cure the longer they stay in the body. If this model were accurate, then doctors could improve cancer survival rates by catching tumors earlier in their development. A cancer that may not be noticeable or dangerous at present will become so later. It thus pays, under this theory, to remove these earlier forms of cancer that would put the person at risk of death if they were left to develop.

During the period between the world wars, doctors attempted to catch changes in tissue morphology before they even became cancerous. Pathologists started to define precancers like, in breast cancer, lobular carcinoma in situ or ductal carcinoma in situ.[16] These carcinomas are not traditional cancers but cells that have started to change their appearance. They were considered cells that were at an extremely early stage of cancer, on the way toward becoming cancerous. Thus women could get a jump on treating cancer by having such precancerous lesions removed. Here again, medicine treated risk: evaluation occurred before the experience of disease or even the pathological indication of disease in order to prevent a worse form of disease in the future.

Of course, no one would find these kinds of lesions without looking for them, and few women would look for them if there were no symptoms. Catching these cancers early enough required a dedicated search among healthy people. Thus the logic of cancer screening was born. The goal of screening was to examine all seemingly healthy people in the hopes of discovering a cancer precursor or an early-stage tumor. Surgeons could remove the tumor while it was still in an unthreatening state. Screening programs started with Pap smears, a relatively cheap and easy way to screen for potential cervical cancers. Pap smears became widespread by the 1960s.[17] The success of this campaign led to the search for a screening tool for the more common breast cancers, a tool provided by mammograms.[18] Today, all women above a certain age (which is still a matter of debate) are recommended to receive a mammogram. If anything suspicious is found, women are sent on for the more precise diagnosis provided by biopsies, which then lead to treatment. Massive public relations campaigns encouraged screening, leading to a widespread acceptance of screening on the part of the public. From women's cancers like breast and cervical cancer, screening spread to other cancers, like prostate and colon cancer, becoming a normal part of preventive care.

Problems of Prevention

While prevention dominates medicine, many scholars and doctors have challenged both screening and pharmaceutical risk management.[19] Some of these challenges involve deeper disputes over the goals and priorities of medicine that I will engage later in the book. In this chapter, though, I will discuss more pragmatic concerns about these procedures. The most important of these worries is that screening and pharmaceutical risk reduction themselves threaten to bring about illness. There is no intervention that does not bear its own risks. Every medication has possible side effects. Every surgery threatens complications. Even entering a hospital carries health risks. The specter of iatrogenic disease, diseases brought about by medical intervention, hovers over all risk reduction programs.[20]

Cancer screening programs illustrate these problems. Initially, it was thought that through screening, cancer could be caught early enough to be treated and thus many cancer deaths could be avoided. What could be a more obvious course of action to reduce the risk of death than to look for disease? Yet once one takes unintended consequences into consideration, matters become more complicated.[21] For example, treatments for cancer are not benign. Chemotherapy and radiation themselves increase risks of cancer. Surgery to remove tumors causes complications, as well as stress, depression, and disfigurement followed by reconstructive surgery. Even the process of screening carries risks: biopsies are surgeries and mammograms use radiation. Debates over these interventions have led to revisions in screening guidelines, reducing the frequency of screenings and targeting them at narrower age ranges. Given our ignorance and the complexity of the calculations, these revisions have in turn spurred controversy.

For example, a prostate-specific antigen (PSA) test for prostate cancer is a simple blood test.[22] If the test is positive, suggesting cancer, then the patient must decide whether to undergo a biopsy, which is an uncomfortable procedure with side effects.[23] There are many false positives with the PSA test, with one study indicating that 15 percent of patients encounter a false positive result over the course of ten years of screening, meaning that the test indicates a cancer although the patient does not actually have cancer.[24] Even knowing the likelihood of a result being a false positive, it is hard to think of someone rationally avoiding the biopsy when he becomes aware of the now greater possible risk of cancer. The first decision to have the PSA test almost forces the second decision to have a biopsy if anything appears. Yet prostate biopsies are not completely benign procedures, with 1 percent of them ending in complications requiring hospitalization. The quest for safety itself leads to risk. Even if the patient goes ahead with the biopsy and gets the relief of a negative result, then the patient still has a greater likelihood of future biopsies and possibly greater anxiety. In all likelihood, there will be greater surveillance and fear even with a good biopsy result.

If the biopsy is positive, then a whole host of possible scenarios open themselves to the patient. He can choose to take a wait and see approach, exercising increased vigilance over the development of the possible cancer, although this almost ensures ongoing anxiety. Treatment options, depending on the stage, include surgical removal of the prostate, radiation therapy, or chemotherapy. Treatment would seem to offer the salvation from death that motivated the initial embrace of the PSA test. Yet it does not. None of the treatments for prostate cancer are 100 percent effective, so there remains the chance of failure. Even if the cancer is declared to be in remission after treatment, the patient is not safe. Because of the ever-present threat of recurrence, he will have to live a life marked by medical surveillance (increased testing), self-surveillance (does that lump indicate anything?), and anxiety.

Moreover, there are risks that he must weigh about the treatment options for prostate cancer. Each brings its own possibilities for suffering. Most can cause impotence and incontinence. Radiation and chemotherapy can even cause secondary cancers that result from their mutagenic effects on cells. Each of these possibilities bring new scenarios and dangers in their train. How will impotence affect his marriage? How will he deal with incontinence? All of these possible futures are bundled into this first moment of decision to have a screening test, as once a train of therapeutic intervention is set in motion, there is no going back.[25]

Even medications that, unlike interventions for cancer, have relatively few side effects may become dangerous once integrated into the risk reduction paradigm. Debates rage over the exact side effects of the statins that address cardiovascular risk, for example.[26] Lowering blood pressure too much can lead to falls among older adults. Medication to address bone density loss can itself cause bone degeneration. Even if the individual drugs are fairly safe, people can be on multiple risk-reducing medications at the same time. The numbers vary by age, with 36.5 percent of eighteen- to forty-four-year-olds on a prescription, 69.6 percent of those aged forty-five to sixty-four, and 90 percent of those over sixty-five.[27] With that many medications, the risk of drug interactions increases, so it becomes difficult to ensure that the doctor's intervention does no harm. One can try a cost/benefit or benefit/burden analysis, but few studies are done on such drug interactions, and frequently the effects are patient specific. Moreover, in systems this complex the calculations quickly spin out of control.

Through these interventions, the patient is made aware of disease, or at least of disease risk, becoming existentially uneasy. Therapy is started, driving the patient further into the experience of disease. Side effects of therapy can even lead to iatrogenic diseases. Here the framework of prevention can anticipate disease by bringing it about. Because of these added risks, many prevention programs have very small effects on rates of all-cause mortality, even if they may prevent death from a specific disease. A recent large-scale study of the efficacy of screening colonoscopies indicated no statistically significant improvement in survival.[28] Similarly, a recent meta-analysis of statins saw relatively modest gains in all-cause mortality, with an absolute risk reduction of .35 percent over six years.[29] Commentators have questioned even this small benefit, though, because the study showed no significant reduction in cardiovascular deaths.[30] If statins do not save lives by preventing cardiovascular deaths, how are they reducing mortality? Perhaps the best evidence of the limits of prevention is the large body of research that has shown that the centerpiece of a preventive health program, the yearly checkup, where all the bloodwork is taken and the screenings are scheduled, has little effect on disease or mortality.[31]

TREATING THE POPULATION

Another problem with the focus on risk is that in this model of medicine the patient receives care that will not necessarily help her as an individual.[32] The data all come from an analysis of the population, which may obscure distinctive features of any individual case. For example, screening programs are still based largely on the idea that all cancers show a similar natural history, developing from relatively benign to metastatic forms. Yet there is disagreement over the natural histories of cancers. From the beginning of the debates over the introduction of mammograms, a number of researchers postulated that many of the newly identified cancers grew slowly, so they would not be a threat during a person's lifetime or at least for many years.[33] Prostate cancer itself can be either aggressive, leading to an early death, or relatively slow-growing, so slow in fact that it would not threaten the man's life unless he lived far beyond average life expectancy. One meta-analysis looked at postmortem studies that histologically examined the prostates of hundreds of men aged seventy to seventy-nine for cancer. These studies found what would be diagnosed on biopsy as prostate cancer in 36 percent of Caucasian Americans and 51 percent of African Americans.[34] These were men who died not of prostate cancer but from other causes. These findings suggest that a large number of older men live for many years with forms of prostate cancer in a way that does not jeopardize their lives. Such findings raise the question of how many cancers are treated that would never have threatened the phenomenological health of the patient. On the other hand, one might ask whether detecting aggressive cancer actually benefits the individual patient if there are few treatment options. These fundamental questions are obscured when looking at population-level statistics.

The question of individual benefit for population-level interventions is even more urgent with regard to risk-reducing pharmaceuticals. Since it is risk rather than actual disease being treated, not everyone will benefit from medications treating risk, like statins. This idea is captured in the concept of number needed to treat (NNT). The NNT is the number of people who would need to take a medication over a certain period of time to have one patient for whom it had its desired effect. Thus, for an effective curative drug like an antibiotic, the NNT is generally fairly low; nearly every person treated with it is cured of their infection. For a preventive medication, the NNT to save a life or prevent a bad outcome will be much higher, generally in the dozens if not hundreds, since only a certain number of individuals taking the medication would have otherwise suffered an adverse event. For example, 286 healthy people need to take a statin for primary prevention, meaning that they did not have a diagnosed disease, to prevent one death.[35] While the appropriate NNT can be debated, the real problem is that the current system of research and drug approval incentivizes pharmaceutical companies to design clinical trials in order to give the largest NNT possible.[36] The more people for whom a drug can be said to significantly (in the statistical sense) reduce risk, even if the absolute risk reduction is quite small, the more prescriptions are written and the more profits the company will make. For these reasons, research is designed to deliver the maximal NNT. Thus the paradigm of risk reduction tied to our current model of financing drug development may actually be giving us less efficient medication, or less efficient guidelines for prescribing medications. Moreover, research has shown that industry-funded studies have a greater tendency to support the products than those not funded by industry.[37]

— This concern with the population is part of the way that the body disappears. Attention is redirected away from the concrete needs of the particular body confronting the doctor to the potential danger threatening the body as envisioned as a member of the population. In risk-based preventive medicine, the focus shifts in two ways, both from present to future and from individual to population. Caring for the population does not always end well for the individual patient. Instead, a preoccupation with future risk can bring ill health in the moment due to side effects. Precision medicine seeks to address some of these concerns by further specification of the population to which a patient belongs so that risk prediction can be more individualized. But as chapter 4 will show, the problems of relating an individual to a population remain even with greater technical precision. Before exploring these tools, though, we must examine how the shift to the population is intimately tied to a second thrust of the paradigm of prevention, genetic risk, which is the topic of the next chapter.

THREE

Genetics and Risk

The company Genomic Prediction promises to reveal a child's future to her parents. If a couple is undergoing IVF, the fertility clinic can select a cell from each of the developing embryos and send them to the company for sequencing.[1] Genomic Prediction offers tests for many of the risks discussed in the last chapter, such as hypertension, coronary artery disease, breast cancer, skin cancer, and prostate cancer, as well as diabetes and schizophrenia. They even considered offering tests for height and intelligence. As you might suspect, these are not tests that will tell the child's exact IQ or whether they will surely have heart disease. Instead, the tests predict risk: in what part of a population the child's likelihood for a condition will fall. How much more susceptible to heart disease than average will this child be? In what quintile of the population is this child's IQ likely to be? The tests predict relative risks, which are comparative numbers. Still, parents are willing to compare their embryos and implant only the ones with the best odds for health and success when compared to the population at large. Under the guidance of a risk paradigm, parents reframe their experiences in terms of fear of hidden dangers. These tests on embryos mirror genetic tests available for the broader public through direct-to-consumer (DTC) sequencing companies as well as emerging clinical uses of genomics in precision medicine.

As these examples show, today's preventive medicine does not just examine physiological indicators. Instead, it looks for a deeper truth, the truth in the genes. Practitioners of precision medicine believe that a more accurate prediction of risk is found in one's DNA, revealing risks that will not appear in physiological indicators until significantly later in the person's life. DNA has long held a fascination in our society as "the Book of Life," or "the Language of Life," the true version of oneself.[2] That is not what DNA is, but as people envision themselves in terms of risk, genetics is assuming this larger role.

This chapter will explore the long history of genetics' obsession with risk. From its origins, genetics sought the true causes of physical disease, mental illness, and social dangers in heredity, a quest that continues today. It has done so through two different approaches, either a focus on the population or a focus on the individual. For the most part, the influence of heredity on the risk of traits appears only in population-level statistics; so genetics, for much of its history, has analyzed comparative risks in populations. Because of this focus, genetics was the field from which most of our statistical tools arose. This population focus is frequently obscured in popular understandings of genetics because of a separate strand of Mendelian genetics that concerned itself with discrete traits as well as the recent success of molecular genetics in relation to a few rare diseases caused by single mutations. The manipulation of discrete traits in an individual is an important aspect of the history of genetics but represents only one paradigm of genetic medicine. Both population- and individual-level genetics, however, have largely attended to preventing disease or unwanted traits, with a focus on genetic cures appearing only late and sporadically. Though the ethics literature primarily addresses issues surrounding genetic manipulations that cure disease, such as CRISPR, the balance of the field today is directed at assessing risk. In its obsession with risk, contemporary genetics reinforces the Gnostic suspicion of the body discussed in chapter 1 by suggesting new loci of danger.

Suspicion of the Population

The field that became genetics arose in part out of fears over the health of the population. The concept of the population was fairly new in the nineteenth century, arising in tandem with the discipline of statistics.[3] In the late eighteenth century, European states had begun to gather more and more data about their societies (births, deaths, production, etc.) in an attempt to develop greater control.[4] As mathematicians began examining these datasets, they discovered surprising regularities. Certain averages would stay nearly constant from year to year: crime, dead letters, even suicides, as Durkheim so famously discussed. These regularities led statisticians to postulate an entity, the population, that displayed these features. A population is therefore a hypothetical construct made up of many individuals that displays regularities over time. Exactly why the population was so regular was unclear, leading to many proposed explanations. Adolphe Quetelet, for example, believed that each nation approximated an *homme moyen*, a national ideal type of height, weight, intelligence, and so forth, that embodied the national average. Quetelet postulated that individuals would diverge from this national ideal type according to mathematical error theory along a normal curve. Some scholars suggested roots for these regularities in cultures, others in sociological structures. Later theorists, the ones we are interested in, would explain regularities through a constant gene pool.

Fears arose as people began to suspect that these population-level regularities were changing for the worse. For example, asylums, as public institutions, collected and reported data on admissions and cures as part of their bureaucratic oversight. The number of people in asylums rapidly rose throughout the nineteenth century.[5] Crime, poverty, and similar social ills also seemed to climb over the course of the century. People, especially members of the professional middle class,[6] sought theories and tools that would help them understand and control these apparent problems, searching for hidden reasons within the body politic for ill health. Many scholars turned to theories that suggested hereditary flaws, views that would lead to eugenics.[7] Some people embraced racist theories that warned of the danger of racial intermixing. Other scholars posited more general theories of hereditary degeneration, arguing that bloodlines declined over time if not carefully tended. After Darwin published his theory of natural selection, some commentators saw the problem as a relaxing of selective pressures in modern society, suggesting that charitable and social welfare institutions allowed too many of the unfit to survive and reproduce. Such ideas led to eugenic policy suggestions, such as the segregation and forced sterilization of those deemed unfit, and ultimately the genocidal policies of the Nazis.[8]

To move beyond broad speculations, scientists sought analytical tools to discover biological mechanisms for social problems. It was Francis Galton, Darwin's cousin, who provided these tools, including the basic concepts of eugenics and statistics. Galton envisioned a pool of hereditary characters that are passed on from one generation to another.[9] He also began gathering data on family lines, trying to determine mechanisms of transmission of traits like intelligence. To analyze these data, he created central concepts in statistics like correlation and regression. Karl Pearson, Galton's biographer and protégé, systematized and further developed Galton's insights.[10] Pearson was the one who, through his management of eugenics and biometrics laboratories and the founding of the journal *Biometrika*, built the scientific infrastructure that led to statistics becoming its own discipline.[11] His field of biometrics sought to better characterize the traits of populations insofar as they were hereditarily derived. To do so, he collected huge amounts of data from asylums and other institutions for eugenic analysis. It was Pearson whose endeavors gave us the tools to interrogate the population.

Yet Pearson envisioned few possibilities for curing the defects that he discovered in the population. Populations are complex, and he wanted to have a far greater understanding of heredity before recommending policies, which is why he never gave official support to the immediate practical implementation of eugenic measures like forced sterilization (although he never opposed such policies either).[12] Part of the reason for his hesitancy was that he hearkened back to an older idea of how characteristics arise. Before scientists emphasized heredity, natural philosophers tended to envision development as the unfolding of the specific potentialities of an individual organism due to that organism's parents and environment.[13] Similarly, Pearson emphasized what he called a diathesis, a set of individual tendencies and potentialities that made up an organism.[14] These were more like general risks and probabilities than determinate traits. Because of the uncertainty of how they might unfold, it was hard to control them. The complexity of heredity suggested to Pearson that population changes occurred slowly over time, as in Darwin's theory. It was difficult to translate population-level insights to the individual.

Statistical Disputes with Mendelians

With the rediscovery of Mendel's work, an alternative to the population-level, probabilistic understanding of traits appeared. Though he wrote his most important paper in 1866, Mendel's work was not broadly appreciated until it was rediscovered by three biologists in 1900.[15] In his focus on the hybridization of different plant varieties, Mendel postulated distinct unit characters for particular traits. This connection of particular traits to single genes, as the unit characters became called, revolutionized discussions of heredity. Rather than a diathesis, a tendency, scientists could discuss a solid causal determinant.

Researchers rapidly found a number of these deterministic traits in humans and other model organisms, leading to what we now know as classical genetics. Some eugenicists then generalized this framework, suggesting that all of the negative traits in the population were caused by single genes. For example, many eugenicists described single traits like feeble-mindedness. Feeble-mindedness was defined as a trait that made the individual incapable of fulfilling his "duties as a member of society in the position of life to which he is born" and that led to many other social ills.[16] Drawing on data from Henry Goddard, many geneticists accepted a heredity narrative for feeble-mindedness into the 1930s.[17] If such negative characteristics were caused by single genes, it would seemingly argue for the effectiveness of eugenicist policy prescriptions such as sterilizing the feeble-minded. Sterilization would prevent this single trait from being transmitted to the next generation.

Pearson's biometric researchers rejected this generalized Mendelian vision. While Pearson accepted that some traits were inherited in a Mendelian fashion, he thought that most of his population-level findings were too complicated to explain in such a determinist way. This led to a long-running battle between Mendelians, led by Gregory Bateson and Charles Davenport, and biometricians.[18] For example, Pearson published an article by David Heron that savagely critiqued Mendelian research on feeble-mindedness. There was a stalemate as to whether to envision heredity in terms of individual determinants or population-level probabilities. Examples could be found for both theories.

In truth, these were not contradictory explanations. One merely had to accept that certain traits were caused by the contributions of multiple

Mendelian genes. Already in 1904, George Udny Yule had shown that the Mendelian and biometric viewpoints could be reconciled, although the acceptance of this reconciliation did not occur until the work of R. A. Fisher, Sewall Wright, and J. B. S. Haldane from 1916 to 1930.[19] These works heralded the birth of population genetics.

These synthetic works created difficulties for the eugenics program. It would be nearly impossible to remove traits from a population through sterilization if they were caused by multiple genes. Even if they were caused by a single recessive gene, the mathematical tools of population genetics, like the Hardy-Weinberg equilibrium, showed that they could not be eliminated by sterilizing only those affected. The genes would remain in heterozygous carriers, destined to reemerge. Some genetic diseases, like sickle cell anemia, are even beneficial in the heterozygous state. Eliminating them would require massive numbers of sterilizations, or at least a commitment to a long campaign over many generations.[20] There would be no simple policy solution to the dangers lurking in the population.

Because of these intellectual difficulties, the horrors of Nazism, and other social pressures against eugenics, eugenics ceased to be a viable political movement for enacting social policies. Instead, it retreated to other areas, such as family and genetic counseling, in which members of the eugenics movement acted at the level of the individual family to prevent the birth of those they deemed unfit.[21] In terms of scientific research, population genetics developed as an important subfield of evolutionary biology, but usually disconnected from social goals.[22] Even those scientists, like sociobiologists, who did address social questions rarely offered much in terms of solutions, seeing fundamental limits to how social programs could transform biologically based problems.[23]

Molecular Genetics

Though population genetics largely stopped directly engaging human characteristics and politics in the mid-twentieth century, the investigation of individual genetic diseases continued under the aegis of molecular genetics. The Rockefeller Foundation launched a major research initiative in the 1930s to investigate the molecular mechanisms of life.[24] It was this program that gave rise to most of the aspects of genetics discussed in bioethics over the last fifty years, like genetic engineering. This research program initiated a major change of scale for biology and heredity, moving from the level of individual people and visible organisms to the level of bacteria, viruses, proteins, and finally DNA. It revolutionized our understanding of biology and medicine.[25]

Molecular genetics is important for my argument because of the way that it reenvisioned development as far more deterministic and mechanistic than Pearson's diathesis. This deterministic approach allowed for the eventual application of population statistics to the management of the individual. Molecular genetics was reductionist, reducing biological problems to their molecular constituents. Already, Thomas Hunt Morgan's *Drosophila* research program had mapped mutations causing single fly traits to determinate positions on chromosomes. Molecular biologists took the next step to connect these genes on a one-to-one basis with enzymes. Using the fungus *Neurospora* as a model, George Beadle found that each mutation he studied blocked a single step in an enzymatic process, suggesting that each gene coded for an enzyme.[26] "One gene, one enzyme" became the watchword. This implied one gene, one trait, marking a move back to the unit factor analysis held by early Mendelians.

This reductionism took the particular form of cybernetics and information theory, as the use of the term genetic *code* suggests.[27] Geneticists viewed organic molecules as containers for information. This information could be transferred through a chain of organic molecules (e.g., from DNA to RNA) governed by feedback and feed-forward loops. Given the hierarchical nature of early cybernetics, this reductionist framework contributed to a genetic determinist vision. As the so-called Central Dogma of molecular biology held, information flowed from DNA to RNA to proteins, and then was presumably translated into traits. Molecular genetics thus led to a reductionist, determinist vision, with genes deterministically giving rise to particular proteins that would engage in molecular processes that determined an organism's characteristics.

This model works for many traits and diseases. In many cases, the segments of DNA that make up a gene are translated into the proteins that are the building blocks of the body, the components that make cells function. If a gene is mutated, then a person is in danger of losing a structural or functional component of the body. This is the basis of many rare genetic diseases like hemophilia, in which proteins necessary for blood clotting are lost because of genetic mutations. Less tragically, there may be distinct forms of a protein encoded by different gene variants, leading to the different blood types, for example. Thus there are some basic cases in which genetic determinism is clearly true.[28]

Molecular genetics also suggests ways to address genetic diseases. One strategy continues the selective strategy of the eugenicists but at the scale of the person.[29] Instead of eugenic sterilization, this strategy encourages the selective abortion of children with genetic diseases. Genetic testing allows for the early identification of these children in the womb or in IVF procedures before implantation. This strategy would prevent disease by preventing the existence of those who would suffer it.[30] The other strategy aims at cure. Researchers seek to correct mutated DNA sequences, returning the affected person to health.[31] Genetic therapy faced disappointment after disappointment for decades, but now, because of new gene editing technologies such as CRISPR/Cas9, these efforts are finally bearing fruit in approved therapies. CRISPR is a technique that allows for a fairly targeted cut at a single location in the genome.[32] While promising treatments for a few single-gene disorders, such as sickle cell anemia, CRISPR probably will not provide many therapies for common diseases. What is notable for this book, though, is that neither the strategy of selection nor that of genetic cure addresses populations or probabilistic thought, as precision medicine and preventive health do. Instead, by the 1980s and 1990s, genetics was almost completely focused on finding cures for felt individual human diseases. However, this project would hit a roadblock exactly at the moment of its seeming triumph, the Human Genome Project.

Toward Precision Medicine

The Human Genome Project looked to be the fulfillment of the molecular genetic research program. It was a massive international project that sequenced the entire human genome, allowing data analysts to identify all human genes. By determining every gene, it sought to give us the key, not only to disease, but to many other aspects of the person. It would find every gene that determined the person's traits, especially genes connected to disease, translating the Book of Life and giving scientists the resources for ever-greater control over human life and society. Then a funny thing happened. The genome was sequenced, and everything turned out to be much more complicated than it had first appeared. When the genome project started, researchers estimated that humans would have something like one hundred thousand genes. They found that we actually have only around twenty thousand to twenty-five thousand genes. At the time, I was an undergraduate researcher in a genetics lab, and I remember the shock that many researchers felt when these initial findings were announced. This is the same number of genes as the nematode worm *C. elegans*, meaning that humans achieve immensely more complexity and capability with approximately the same number of genes. Thus there cannot be any one-to-one gene-trait correspondence. Instead, much depends on how these genes are regulated and how they interact, meaning that there is a lot of flexibility in how the genome determines our traits.

Of course, there were many in the field of genetics to whom this finding was not a surprise. Geneticists have long known that for many traits a certain genotype does not lead invariably to a phenotype, a phenomenon known as incomplete penetrance. Population geneticists have known that many traits are caused by the interaction of a number of genes, or pleiotropy. It has also long been known that environmental factors and even personal history influence some traits through mechanisms like epigenetics. What was new after the genome project was that developments pushed this knowledge from the fringes of the field to the center. These phenomena ceased to be interesting but minor exceptions to a largely determinist picture and became central to our understanding of genetics.

Moreover, research in many fields of genetics was showing that genes did not necessarily determine a trait but merely increased the likelihood of that trait. For example, people theorized that many cancers were caused by mutations that happen over a lifetime in response to everyday mutagens, such as ultraviolet light hitting the skin, cigarette smoke affecting the lung, or even just the random errors that occur when copying DNA. These kinds of mutations are stochastic, meaning that they happen unpredictably and by chance at the individual level, but the rates of mutation can be predicted at the population level. Most heritable cancer-causing mutations lie in genes for fixing these mistakes or in genes regulating cell proliferation. Rather than determining cancer, heritable cancer-causing mutations became predispositions to cancer.[33] The extent of the predisposition can be measured statistically.

Other developments occurred outside the field of genetics to push a new paradigm. As the last chapter discussed, driven by the success of the Framingham Heart Study, medicine began to shift its focus away from felt illness or deterministic causes of disease like infectious agents to risk factors for disease. Genes began to be thought of along the lines of these risk factors; geneticists saw them as predisposing the person to certain diseases. As they discovered that there were not many genes that caused a major predisposition to disease, geneticists started to look for smaller increases in risk, or combinations of genes that were risk factors. This is a very different mode of thought from genetic determinism.

Finally, movements entirely outside medicine and biomedical science affected this new understanding of genetics. For twenty years now, tech companies have sought to design algorithms that sweep up the massive amounts of information provided on the internet and use it to sell products: tailor searches, target ads, recommend things you might like, and so on.[34] These algorithms are based on statistical correlations revealed by large datasets. This Big Data approach has spread to many other fields like parole board recommendations, election strategy, and news delivery, to name a few. For the last twenty years, this same approach has been central to genetics because the genome is such a massive dataset. At a very early stage of the genome project, genome centers and genetics labs began recruiting programmers who were trained in the tech industry's Big Data paradigm to help them interpret genomic information.[35] The overlap is becoming even greater as many tech companies move into the field of healthcare, directly providing analytics and wearable health devices.[36] These analytics use data to predict health risk.

Thus the field of genetics has become committed to the idea that hereditary traits emerge through the interaction of many genes and stochastic mutations, acting as risk factors rather than determinant causes, in a way that can be analyzed only through intensive computational methods, leading to a new framework for human genetics. It is still a cybernetic, reductionist account of the person, merely not a deterministic one. This framework hearkens back to the probabilistic focus on population found in Pearson's work, but in a way that harmonizes with the emphasis on health risks in preventive medicine. Most importantly, this new way of envisioning genetics allows Pearson's concerns over population risk to be directly translated to the individual patient. Genetics seeks to quantify the individual's risk of various diseases by identifying him with a particular subpopulation.

This turn to individual risk interpreted through information on the population can be seen in new analyses of Polygenic Risk Scores (PRSs), the central tool of the emerging field of precision medicine.[37] Given the limitations of single-gene analyses, geneticists asked whether they could predict risks due to the combined action of many genes. They use a technique called a "genome-wide association study" that examines thousands of DNA sites across the genome that differ between people.[38] These sites vary in a single DNA base pair, with the variants called single nucleotide polymorphisms (SNPs). Basically, what geneticists do is take thousands of people, measure a trait like height, intelligence, or diabetes, and see whether each variant of a SNP is correlated with the trait and how much it contributes to the risk of that trait. They find associations with a trait in genes located across the genome. By adding up all the increased and decreased risks across the genome, researchers quantify a PRS, the risk that a person will have a trait. So for heart disease, a person who had many SNPs correlated with increased risk of heart attack would be at high risk for the disease. There would be other people who would be low risk because of their specific SNPs not being associated with heart disease risk. Note that this is *risk*, not determinism.

Despite problems with PRS that chapter 4 will discuss, genomic tools like it are becoming integrated into preventive medicine. Precision medicine seeks to exploit the tie between genetics and risk by identifying every individual risk factor. Now, the person is not safe merely because she does not have a major genetic mutation. Instead, she is always at risk due to the thousands of small risk factors that lie in her genome. By alerting consumers to them, DTC sequencing companies are driving these risks into the public imagination. Established medicine seeks to join in the surveillance of risk through research programs like the All of Us project described earlier. This synergy is no coincidence. Preventive medicine and predictive genetics both emerge from a paradigm emphasizing risk and populations;

genetics just gets at a deeper level of prediction than can be found in physiological markers or scans.

Reductionism and the Population

Many philosophical and theological critiques of genetics take aim at its reductionism. Genetic explanations can reduce the rich complexity of human life to deterministic outcomes of a gene or a network of genes. Genetic determinism thus obscures the effects of culture, history, language, thought, and free will in human action and human characteristics.[39] Reductionism becomes especially dangerous when the person is identified with a single gene that leads to congenital disease, leading to selection against him. These are all serious dangers that come from interpreting human life in terms of heredity.

Yet this determinism is not the only or even the oldest possibility for thinking about heredity's relationship to human society. Rather, it is only one historical modality of interpreting heredity. The determinist, reductionist vision of genetics that simplistically ties human actions to a few traits arose through the efforts of the early twentieth-century Mendelian eugenicists, especially in the United States, and then receded with the rise of population genetics. Deterministic understandings of heredity again became a dominant strand of thought through the success of molecular genetics. It was in this form that the earliest bioethicists encountered genetics in the 1970s through the 1990s, and wrestling with genetic determinism still dominates many bioethical arguments about genetics.

Before the rediscovery of Mendel, there was a very different interpretation of heredity, one that focused on populations. The population paradigm does not pronounce determinisms but rather speaks in terms of propensity, diathesis, and probability. It eschews mechanistic analyses of causality (Gene A leads to Trait B) but instead embraces a positivism dependent on large datasets that are almost uninterpretable in terms of traditional biological mechanisms.[40] This population approach to heredity arose early with Galton and Pearson and survived the Mendelian challenge by mutating into population genetics. This vision dominates most genetic research in the post–Human Genome Project world.

While its eschewal of determinism is to be welcomed, it still raises a host of ethical issues that are as yet underexplored and undertheorized. Though avoiding determinism, it allows for a statistical reduction of the person to the data of risk. If genetic determinism unalterably fixes the individual person in a certain form, the population perspective tends to cause the individual person to disappear. She is seen in terms of her position on a number of normal curves describing population-level characteristics. The individual body, as it exists in the present, ceases to be of much concern, as this framework looks to probabilities for the future. Understanding heredity in terms of population thus fits well with the paradigm of prevention that ignores the concrete sensations of the individual body.

Moreover, viewing individuals in terms of the population, although not as damaging as pigeonholing them into a particular outcome, is not free of danger. As eugenics showed, understanding society in terms of populations can still lead to the destruction of human life. It too is imbued with the suspicion of bodies and the fear of hidden dangers, only in terms of the population as a whole. It demands that we consider the risks present in ourselves and the possible risks in our children's genes. Probabilistic accounts of human capabilities still lead to the selective destruction of the human person, as with the services of the Genomic Prediction company described in the opening of the chapter. Moreover, this population-level vision fits well with other kinds of managerial paradigms that aim at controlling human life. There is a more basic problem to examine first, though, that of correlating individuals and populations.

FOUR

Individuals and Populations

The pharmaceutical company Medco was disappointed with the results of the clinical trial for what would become the drug BiDil,[1] which is a combination of two generic drugs meant to treat high blood pressure. Unfortunately for the company, the clinical trial showed that a new drug class of angiotensin-converting enzyme inhibitors was more effective than its generic drug combination. Further, the results for BiDil's effectiveness were not statistically significant. Desperate to salvage something from this study, researchers reanalyzed the data, using multiple statistical techniques and methods of segmenting the population of research subjects. Eventually, they found that if they isolated the results for Black patients in the trial, they saw a statistically significant positive result. On the basis of these data and a follow-up trial in Black patients, BiDil became the first drug approved for a specific racial group.

Many scholars decried this approval because there seemed to be no logic for why the medication should specifically work for Black patients. First, race is not a meaningful biological category, as geneticists have argued for decades; there is more genetic diversity within racial groups than between them.[2] Race is, of course, an important *social* category, with implications for socioeconomic status and treatment by others, but social identity should not affect the biological response to a pharmaceutical agent. Thus there is no plausible mechanism as to why a drug would work better in one racial group than another. Second, many statisticians criticized the way the reanalysis segmented the population. Reanalyzing results until one gets a positive finding is pejoratively called torturing the data. Given the size of clinical trials, researchers can always find some type of correlation or significant difference between groups in a dataset given enough time and effort. The problem is that most of these associations will be spurious. For example, a reanalysis was able to "prove" a statistically significant correlation between not drinking and risk of heart disease that held only for those born under the astrological signs of Capricorn and Cancer.[3] That is why best practice is to describe the statistical analysis that will be used before executing the clinical trial (a process called preregistration).[4] Both of these concerns regard whether the right population was chosen for analysis and treatment (i.e., whether a racial group is a biologically meaningful population and whether the statistical analysis properly segmented a population). Determining whether a proper population is chosen, however, is a much broader problem of preventive medicine.

The last chapters discussed the mistakes that could be made when the individual person is seen only in terms of statistics. Even from a purely medical or biostatistical perspective, the new technologies of risk analysis and precision medicine raise dangers of misrecognition through failures to acknowledge the difficulties of relating the individual to the population. This chapter explores two problems emerging from genomic research that tries to predict risk. The first regards whether the analysis has used the right population for its sample, especially when the practitioner applies the results to the individual patient. The second regards the broader question of how to apply group-level information to any individual. Broadly, the chapter will explore issues of individuals and populations.

Before beginning this discussion, though, it is important to make a brief note about terminology. The categories used in the genetics and health literature are not always used in a standardized way, leading to confusion as to whether authors intend a social group, a group sharing genetic ancestry, or a geographical group. Even terms as basic as *ancestry* or *population* can have multiple meanings.[5] Things get much more complicated when using terms such as *race* or *ethnicity*. Here I will use *race* to distinguish a social category. There is no necessary connection between socially ascribed race and any biological population. I will use the term *descent* to distinguish a group with some sort of presumed shared genetic ancestry or at least genetic similarity due to a historically limited geographical range.

This is not a perfect set of distinctions by any means. Moreover, descent groups should not be reified as distinct entities because they share many genetic characteristics with other groups and there has always been intermarriage between nearby populations. Some natural population groups do have some common genetic features, usually historically geographically isolated populations. For example, Iceland was largely, if not completely, isolated from other interbreeding groups for many hundreds of years and derived from a few founders. For this reason, one of the first large genomic projects, run by deCODE Genetics, used Icelandic DNA.[6] Such groups are rare, though, especially in a country as diverse and intermixed as the United States.

Bias and Populations

One basic problem of contemporary genetics is that genomic and biobank projects have tended to collect their samples from a very restricted population. Most DNA samples historically have come from people of European descent, and, among this group, disproportionately from middle-class, middle-aged women,[7] although this is changing with new programs like the All of Us project that are explicitly seeking greater diversity.[8] Such oversampling of a very restricted population means that any risk predictions derived from these studies probably will not be generalizable. Statistical characteristics, like the risks of heart disease for a certain genetic variant, are highly dependent on the specific population that was analyzed. If you take a risk prediction algorithm derived from the genetic analysis of people of European descent, for example, it probably will not accurately predict risks for people of Korean descent, or even for a mixed population like the one treated by U.S. healthcare. The exact mix of genetic variants will not be the same.

Moreover, the exclusion of minority groups from these studies causes researchers to miss important data. For example, rare variants affecting disease risk may exist in populations of both Icelandic and Igbo descent but perhaps be more common in the Nigerian group. A genetic analysis of a group of Icelandic descent alone may not catch the gene variant's contribution to disease because of its relative rarity in that population, even though it causes significant risk for particular individuals. Thus many geneticists argue that including diverse groups can help improve risk prediction for everyone. Alternatively, a genetic variant may have a distinct effect in a different genetic background due to the interaction with other genetic variants. The overall genetic background of a group of Mayan descent may make a risk caused by a certain gene variant more apparent than will the genetic background of a group of Italian descent. Seeing the genetic variant's effect in different populations can give a much better understanding of how genes function and the risks that they entail. It is thus crucial to diversify the samples for these studies.

There are several reasons why these research samples are fairly homogeneous. The first is just the convenience of collecting samples. The samples of convenience, the people who send their DNA into 23andMe or who initially volunteer for biobank projects, tend to fit a certain demographic: trusting in science, prosperous, and eager to know their risk. These features characterize the upper middle class, which tends not to represent the population as a whole. Researchers have not done enough to broaden their reach, which admittedly takes effort. More recent projects like the NIH's All of Us program are making more concerted efforts at diversity.[9]

A second reason is convenience of analysis. If a population is very heterogeneous, then statisticians need a lot more DNA samples to make meaningful correlations appear. In a group that is relatively homogeneous in both genetic and social terms, the health effects of the few genetic variants will stand out more. A heterogeneous group will have a lot more noise. Researchers must be willing to wrestle with complexity by developing better statistical techniques if they want to engage a diverse sample. Even then, no strong associations may exist in highly mixed populations.

Finally, many people who are racial minorities have not donated samples to these projects because of skepticism with regard to the field of genetics and biomedical research more generally. Minorities are aware of the racism of eugenics described in the last chapter. They also know the history of racial minorities who were exploited in horrifying research projects like the Tuskegee Syphilis Study or whose contributions to science were overlooked, as with HeLa cells.[10] This justified skepticism about the aims, procedures, and ownership of genetic research extends back into the 1990s and before. Overcoming it will require outreach, partnering with civil society groups, a more diverse set of researchers, and a clear commitment to ethical research.[11]

Yet these issues just scratch the surface of the contemporary practice of genetics. There are far more basic methodological problems with relating individual risk to population statistics, especially with regard to race and descent groups.[12] When trying to diversify statistical prediction, researchers can choose to develop either a single polygenic risk score (PRS) for everyone or a PRS specific to each different population, such as each descent group or racial category. A single overall PRS will probably not give much information for the reasons described above; there will be too few significant correlations discovered in a heterogeneous population. Even a racially specific PRS will be misleading because race is not a biological category. It is a social category. Thus, even if researchers were to develop a PRS tailored to a certain race, there is no way to know if a specific patient would actually belong to that group.

For a concrete example of these difficulties, take a research trial on breast cancer screening.[13] The experimental arm of the trial assigned women to different risk groups (high-, average-, and low-risk groups) based on the Breast Cancer Surveillance Consortium (BCSC) risk calculator (which uses standard clinical and physiological measurements to determine risk of breast cancer) as well as their PRS for breast cancer. The control arm used only the BCSC risk calculator. The researchers adjusted screening recommendations according to risk and age (which is another marker of risk), with high-risk women advised to get mammograms much more often than low-risk women. This study succeeded in recruiting a diverse pool of research subjects, and as more data regarding genetic correlations to breast cancer risk in different racial groups appeared they tailored their screening recommendations accordingly. There were specific genetic variants that were included only for certain racial minorities, and the weightings of different SNPs were adjusted according to race. As new data appeared, sometimes women were moved from high- to low-risk.

Anthropologists studying this trial described the case of a woman who was moved into a low-risk group because she self-identified as Hispanic. Faced with a change in risk status, the woman started to doubt whether she had correctly identified herself. Her origins and family were in Spain, and she spoke Spanish, so she considered herself Hispanic. But although she socially identified as Hispanic, she wondered whether her genetic background should be considered European or Hispanic. This question is unanswerable in an objective way because these categories are self-reported rather than based in objective biological data. These kinds of problems with self-identification appeared repeatedly in this study. How to proceed in this analysis is not a trivial problem since the results will determine whether the patient is exposed to increased screening, with its attendant dangers.

Further, any sample is going to be biased by the population from which it was taken, a problem for both a broad PRS and a racially specific PRS. That is the point of sampling; a sample describes only a particular group that was sampled. Even if one looked only at Latin American populations, risk scores derived from a sample from Cuba would be different from ones derived from a sample from Chile, and different samples taken from within Cuba would also be different. All statistical predictions are biased to the population from which they were taken.[14] Thus statistical generalizations will not necessarily be valid for any other group. For this reason, statistical tools are not portable in an unbiased way, unless the population you apply the tool to is exactly the same as the one that was sampled, which is impossible to ensure. Hidden confounders in the population structure will frequently defeat statistical tools. There will always be bias in statistical prediction, but the question is how much is acceptable and what kinds of bias we want. Those are political rather than scientific questions.

From the Population to the Individual

If it is difficult to determine which population to use in an analysis, it is even more challenging to determine how to apply population-level statistics to the individual. The economist Frank Knight divided decisions into those that involved risk and those that involved uncertainty.[15] A person can reliably use statistics on risk when he is making the same decision a large number of times—as when a hospital administrator estimates readmissions by predicting how many surgeries will have complications. He can predict the general number of readmissions based on past experience and set aside the appropriate resources to deal with them. This works at the level of a general aggregate.

Any singular decision, however, will be made under what Knight calls conditions of uncertainty, for which there is no sure quantitative measure.[16] Even if the hospital administrator might know how many complications there will be across hundreds of surgeries, neither the surgeon nor the patient knows whether in *this individual case* there will be a complication. Population statistics give only a general sense. That is why most decision theorists characterize probabilistic decision-making in individual cases as akin to gambling.[17] The person is making a bet on the likelihood of an outcome. Statistics on risk are more like the odds of a sporting event. While there are better and worse gambling strategies, it is not irrational to bet against the odds, a point that is especially salient as I write these words soon after a horse overcame 80-to-1 odds to win the Kentucky Derby.

The way genetic risk is described in precision medicine makes this clear. Originally, genetics promised a personalized medicine. It swiftly became apparent that genetics would not be able to predict any individual's personalized risk. Instead, it would place them in a stratified risk group.[18] It would tell them whether they were at higher or lower risk for a certain disease than is average in a population. That still leaves a great deal of interpretive work to be done to decide how to apply that risk score to an individual.

Few genetic mutations condemn a person to a disease in a certain and deterministic way. There is variability in how severe many of them are, like cystic fibrosis. The famous breast cancer gene BRCA1 leads only to a predisposition to breast cancer, with an estimated 55 to 72 percent of women with the mutation developing breast cancer as opposed to 13 percent of women in the population at large.[19] Yet women who receive this information will often proceed to quite drastic preventive measures, like prophylactic double mastectomies. With increased genetic sequencing and newborn screening, we are seeing more and more variability in outcomes.

Even broader genetic analysis reveals only so much about risk. A PRS is quite limited in its predictive value for individuals. Even the best of the current PRSs rarely predicts much over 10 percent of the variance in a trait. That leaves most of the variability in a population unexplained. Moreover, there is a tremendous variability even within people sharing a risk score. Let's say that a person's PRS for a disease put him in the eightieth percentile of risk; people within that group will still show a broad distribution of outcomes, describing a broad bell curve. In fact, the outcomes of many people at high risk will overlap with those of many people at low risk, which raises questions of what such scores really tell us.

When the great evolutionary biologist Stephen Jay Gould was diagnosed with mesothelioma, an incurable cancer, in 1982, he discovered that the median survival for patients with the disease was only eight months. Thankfully for his state of mind, he had worked enough with statistics to know that population-level descriptions of statistical data do not necessarily mean anything for an individual. "All evolutionary biologists know that variation itself is nature's only irreducible essence. Variation is the hard reality.... Means and medians are the abstractions,"[20] as are all PRSs. He considered his individual characteristics and decided that they would likely place him in the longer-lived portion of the group with the disease. In the end, his doubts about the hard reality of statistical predictions were correct. He lived for twenty years after his diagnosis.

— There is no answer as to how to apply risk information to the individual. It is even difficult to know which sorts of risk predictions are founded on the proper dataset for any particular person because of the problem of fitting them to the right population. The individual body cannot disappear into the population. We are faced with the basic choice of how much risk is acceptable, a choice we will discuss again in chapter 6. Enthusiasts of preventive medicine will embrace a higher NNT and a greater level of intervention, accepting a population perspective. However, more interventions will generate their own risks. The individual is always making decisions under uncertainty, even with the most thorough statistical analysis. The questions at play are more ethical than scientific. Yet as the next chapter will discuss, bioethics as a field has intensified the focus on population management in medicine without addressing these questions.

FIVE

Public Health Ethics and Clinical Ethics

Over the last fifty years, bioethics has transformed medicine, serving as a critical check on the expansion of medical power over the patient. Some ethicists sought to empower the patient through a more individualistic emphasis on patient autonomy and informed consent. Other bioethicists took a more relational approach, encouraging a richer doctor-patient relationship grounded in the virtues of the practitioner. These latter scholars sought to recover an older clinical ethos that risks being deformed by technological medicine. All bioethicists aimed at protecting the individual patient, and the field has made many contributions to this end.

Now, however, elements of medical ethics have begun to embrace the medical focus on the care of the population. Even many religious ethicists are turning toward a population perspective, as seen in Michael Rozier's renarration of the corporal works of mercy in light of population health priorities: "For I was hungry and you ensured I did not live in a food desert, I was thirsty and you guaranteed my tap water was safe to drink, a stranger and your laws allowed me to find asylum, naked and your donation did not shame me, ill and you ensured I had affordable health insurance, in prison and the system rehabilitated me."[1] He admits that his version is not as inspiring as the original and that he finds little support for population health in Christian scripture. But he thinks it necessary, given the current state of knowledge, to reinterpret the corporal works of mercy in terms of population-level interventions. This turn to the social aims at shifting medical ethics from a clinical ethos focused on the individual patient to a public health ethos concerned with the population. Rozier is far from alone in this goal, with many other religious bioethicists encouraging population-level interventions.[2] Secular bioethicists also have long sought to integrate public health policy perspectives into bioethics.[3] These calls to manage the population have only intensified with growing medical attention to health disparities, especially in the aftermath of the Covid-19 pandemic.

Much of this turn to public health ethics may merely indicate that the discipline of bioethics is following medicine in its shift toward prevention described in the last three chapters.[4] Yet there are also reasons internal to bioethics that support this shift. This chapter will describe some historical reasons contributing to ethicists' support for population health. Bioethicists' laudable struggle to reduce paternalism, rein in technology, and support justice paradoxically has led to an institutional control that aims to foster the health of populations rather than necessarily healing individual patients. Despite my commitment to the field of bioethics, I am concerned about this shift. Subsequent chapters will explain why, even if its substantive goals are good, preventive health and precision medicine are false answers to concerns over justice.

The Rise of Bioethics

The first chapter described one version of medical ethics in terms of a clinical ethos in which the doctor professes her desire and ability to help a suffering patient through the technical skills of medicine. This ethical ideal held for much of medicine's history. Even when the patient could not pay, there was a call for the doctor to serve out of love for humanity. Moreover, for most of medical history, each doctor faced fierce competition for patients' fees from other doctors and other sorts of healers, so doctors were forced to attend to the patient's concerns and desires.[5] There were thus both pecuniary and ethical motives for a good relationship with the patient.

Such an ethos was always merely an ideal frequently betrayed in the day-to-day scramble to attract and retain paying clients.[6] Yet ideals of physicians' virtue could still guide training and serve as a ground for critique of current practice. While always an ideal, by the middle of the twentieth century with the advance of technological medicine, the clinical ethos diverged ever further from the reality of even the best doctors.[7] Much of medical care shifted into hospitals, and top doctors were ever more likely to double as researchers. Academic doctors began spending more time treating their patients as research subjects, creating conflicts of interest and leading to terrible research scandals.[8] Medicine became more and more infused with a technological outlook.

Outcries over the changed nature of a medicine that was ever more closely entwined with scientific research led to demands for the ethical regulation of medicine, demands that ultimately gave rise to bioethics.[9] Three concerns of early bioethicists are closely tied to my argument. First, bioethicists rejected the paternalism caused by physicians' monopoly on knowledge and decision-making. Diagnoses may or may not have been shared with the patient according to the doctor's discretion, but decisions on treatment lay solely with the doctor. Second, there was a concern over the reductionism of technological medicine.[10] Technological developments disrupted the tradition of the clinical ethos, since the new molecular biology, new surgeries, and new diagnostics all diminished the centrality of the clinical history. The patient's voice disappeared from the clinic, replaced by the numbers and scans discussed in chapter 2. In reductionist medicine, the body disappears, but in a different way than in population health: the body is fragmented into organ systems, cells, and proteins. The patient's voice disappears with her body. Finally, the expense of the technologies and treatments of the new scientific medicine raised issues of distributive justice.[11] Is it right to spend this much money on a single patient? Given limited resources, which patients should receive care? With deepening government involvement in medicine after the establishment of Medicare and Medicaid, questions of distributive justice became more pressing. These three topics are all closely connected, as the complexity and reductive nature of medicine both gave the doctor a unique epistemic authority while also requiring greater resources.

End-of-life care in the ICU exemplifies the interconnection of concerns over paternalism, reductionism, and justice. The technology of the ICU treats the body as a machine: replacing breathing with the bellows-driven function of the ventilator, externally managing the body's fluid balance, and intervening in other aspects of the body as one would manage a highly complex machine.[12] Doctors were reluctant to give patients or their families any say in discontinuing treatment, frequently failing to give a prognosis and sometimes not even telling patients of a terminal diagnosis, leading to legal challenges seeking the right to withdraw treatment. The expensive maintenance of dying patients raised questions of the reasonableness of the costs. End-of-life care was therefore one of the chief areas in which bioethics pushed back against medicine, with patient advocates seeking a more holistic care for the dying, as would be found in hospice, along with more honesty in communication, autonomous decision-making on the part of the patient, and ways of constraining cost.

Paternalism

Bioethics, and medicine more generally, addressed these three concerns in ways that paved the way for the inroads of preventive medicine and population health. For example, the main response to paternalism was to try to dethrone the authority of the doctor. Patient autonomy became the rallying cry of bioethicists and patient advocates. Rather than doctors making exclusive decisions, patients were to choose the treatment options that best accorded with their values.

In the best of circumstances, a recognition of patient autonomy accentuates the healing relationship through shared decision-making between the practitioner and patient. Through in-depth conversations, the practitioner learns the patient's values and uses that knowledge to help the patient discern which treatment options best align with those priorities. All too frequently, though, the doctor, fearing paternalism, becomes merely a provider of information, listing the risks and benefits of various procedures and leaving it to the patient to figure out an answer.[13] Since patients lack knowledge of these fields and the practical experience to judge treatment options, they feel adrift. Or sometimes practitioners, unable to unilaterally determine treatment, manipulate patients' choices by the way they frame options or by browbeating patients. Alternatively, embracing their autonomy, patients become beholden to other, perhaps less reliable sources for judgment, such as DTC pharmaceutical advertisements or social media.

For these reasons, patient autonomy has failed as a concrete solution to the question of decisional authority in the healing relationship.

In fact, the primary outcome of the attack on medical paternalism has been to shift the locus of authority outside of the healing relationship altogether. Rather than reversing the relative power of doctor and patient, it has caused the doctor's power to become diffused into the healthcare team, which ultimately comes under the authority of healthcare administrators of some sort.[14] This shift has been driven by the changing institutional structure of medicine. Whereas in the 1960s most doctors were in private practice, today most practitioners are employed by health systems, making them employees rather than independent professionals. Thus their decisions can be influenced by institutional priorities. Moreover, today's insurers seek much more influence over treatment decisions. The locus of control in medicine has moved from the healing relationship to the larger institution.

This organizational shift has encouraged preventive medicine. Institutions think primarily in procedural terms, which is why so many practical aspects of patient autonomy concern signing an appropriate document. Institutions also think in terms of statistical populations. As I will discuss in chapter 7, institutions and insurers are seeking to use population metrics to decrease the cost of healthcare and increase its efficiency. They can do so only if they influence treatment decisions in light of population effects. Precision and preventive medicine serve as the perfect vehicles for this task. Insofar as ethicists continue along the antipaternalist line of thought, they tend to embrace these institutional measures. Indeed, many ethicists embracing a public health perspective, like Rozier, point to institutional transformation as a primary reason for making this shift.[15] Yet the phenomenological focus on the patient's bodily health disappears when the primary authority for treatment decisions moves out of the healing relationship and into the institutional realm.

Reductionism

At first glance, antireductionism would seem to support a phenomenological focus on the patient's bodily experience. Early bioethicists criticized mid-twentieth-century medicine for embracing a Cartesian dualism that separated the patient's experience from the bodily machine.[16] Medicine seemed to focus only on curing or physical maintenance rather than on reintegrating the person to make him whole. Scientific medicine neglected the social circumstances, the lived world of the patient, that caused or exacerbated disease. Eric Cassel describes a patient with pneumonia, which was caused by his not eating well and subsequent malnourishment, which in turn was caused by knee pain that prevented him from going shopping, which he did not seek to heal because of a depression brought on by grief over his wife's death and the resulting social isolation.[17] Healing this patient required not only addressing the immediate physiological details of the pneumonia but also physical therapy for the knee, social supports that would help him to get groceries, and ultimately a renewed social world. Medicine cannot provide a social world, but it can at least recognize the problem and encourage solutions. Because illness emerges from the complex interactions of patients' lives, medicine needs to acknowledge the whole and to care for the patient as a person, not just cure the physical body. Care becomes especially important when cure is impossible.

This admirable holism, however, also served to open the door to the perspective of the population. The whole that is the patient's life can be described in different ways. One way involves the qualitative exploration of the individual's social world and its impact on her health. Yet some objective aspects of a patient's social world can also be quantitatively described. The patient's poverty, food insecurity, or access to housing can all be portrayed in statistical terms in relationship to the broader population. The effects of these social factors on health can be probabilistically predicted. These are what became termed the social determinants of health.[18]

An emphasis on social determinants of health can lead to many goods. However, the quantitative description of these social factors is much more amenable to scientific and institutional medicine than a more phenomenological exploration of the specifics of a patient's social world. Social science can be just as reductive as natural science. Again, the person disappears, this time not into the mechanical description of biological processes but into the numerical description of social processes. The patient is again reduced to an abstracted portion of her story that can be quantified. Care then becomes preventive, focused on the future illness predicted by statistics. As bioethics moved into the domain of lawyers, policy experts, and utilitarians, this quantitatively manipulable public health perspective became ever more popular.

JUSTICE

The social determination of disease also highlights important issues of justice. Early bioethical discussions of justice concerned the problem of distribution: How does one distribute a scarce resource, like an organ?[19] Or how much should we pay for expensive end-of-life care when many people lack basic care? Some of these early debates argued over the proper amount to spend on preventive care in contrast to expensive treatments. The debate over distribution grew in importance with rising medical expenditures. As healthcare spending skyrocketed, economists and ethicists sought ways to rein in spending, asking how much we could afford to spend on healthcare in relation to other social goods, like education.

There were two responses to these questions. First, there was the aforementioned public health argument in favor of preventive medicine rather than curative medicine. It is proverbial that an ounce of prevention is worth a pound of cure and a stitch in time saves nine. Thus there has been a turn to pharmaceutical and genetic risk management as a way to restrain spending to the end of a more just distribution of social resources. This is the logic of much of the value-based care and population health policy work that chapter 7 will discuss. The logic of using preventive care to restrain costs is questionable for the pragmatic medical reasons discussed in chapter 2, but it also is unlikely to be economically cost-effective because preventive measures are themselves costly.[20] Even proponents for prevention admit that anyone saved an early death by prevention will probably just end up with a more expensive illness later on.[21]

There is another strategy that totally eschews individuals. If much of ill health is caused by social conditions, such as poverty, then medicine must address these social determinants of health. Medicine's gaze then turns from the individual patient to the conditions of the population that cause disease. The population becomes the patient. There is much to be said for this turn to social conditions, but there are also dangers discussed in the next chapters.

— Forces latent in early bioethics opened the field to the public health ethos, turning it from its original embrace of the clinical ethos. Dethroning medical paternalism empowered institutional actors who thought in terms of populations. Opposition to a reductionist vision of the body as a network of cells and molecules slid into a holism of the population, which can be just as much an objectification of human experience, only through statistical quantification rather than mechanistic description. Confronting injustice caused by high medical expenses leads to cost control through prevention and social change. Everything can shift to risk and population.

This progression was not inevitable. Voices in bioethics called for centering decisions in the intersubjective healing relationship. Other bioethicists developed narrative and holistic frames for capturing more of patients than just their physiology.[22] As we will see in the last part of this book, there are richer ways to investigate health justice than merely looking at a statistically mediated policy framework. These alternatives are still live options.

It is important to continue exploring these other options because a risk-based focus on prevention through population health contains its own dangers. We can question whether medicine is the proper field to determine these questions of social arrangements. Given its possible expansion to all risks and social conditions, it threatens to lead to a totalizing medicalization of life, demanding an increasing amount of control and the exclusion of elements that cannot be controlled. It can undermine a true vision of the other, seeing the patient only in terms of population-level statistics and losing sight of aspects of experience that cannot be quantified. Finally, it raises ever-increasing demands on the individual to care for his life.

Part II

Ethical Problems of Prevention

SIX

The Limitless Demand for Health

The World Health Organization (WHO) defines health as "a state of complete physical, mental and social well-being and not merely the absence of disease or infirmity. The enjoyment of the highest attainable standard of health is one of the fundamental rights of every human being."[1] At first glance, it seems like a beautiful goal, the kind of goal we should seek, until one thinks about the impossibility of its realization. What kind of control would be necessary to achieve this almost limitless health? Many ethicists have criticized the expansiveness of this notion of health,[2] but the full magnitude of this demand becomes apparent only when we understand that many health risks are increasingly understood as diseases in their own right. Perhaps the right to health, then, is a right to be not only free of disease but perhaps even free of risk itself. Such a definition of the right to health sets an endless task. This boundless pursuit of health is inherent to the public health ethos and preventive medicine more broadly.

The breadth of this vision of health suggests the feature of preventive medicine discussed in this chapter: there is no rational bound to the goal of risk reduction. First, every particular risk can always be further reduced. No one is at zero risk for common ailments. Unless a disease is eliminated from the world, like smallpox, its risk can be reduced. Second, we can always consider a broader number of risks. A patient may not be at elevated risk for heart disease, but what about cancer, or Alzheimer's, or kidney failure? Or further, we can consider social sources of health problems: risks of gun violence, food insecurity, and so forth. The field of vision within which to consider risks can always expand. There is no bound to the quantitative reduction of risk.

The limitless nature of preventive medicine also leads to broader problems of political action as discussions around health risks overtake other ways of addressing social issues. As the WHO constitution and many other documents suggest, there is a right to medical care. As a right, it is a political issue. Even when considered only under the guise of curative treatment, a right to healthcare has been difficult to secure. This right becomes much more demanding when health is described in terms of risk. Given finite resources, there are only so many risks a nation can address. How do we choose between them? Even risks that nations do confront can only be reduced so far, so how do we determine the acceptable level of risk? Moreover, by reducing one risk, a program will create other risks, since, as chapter 2 described, every effort at risk reduction will have side effects. What kind of side effects are acceptable? Because there are no rational limits to risk reduction, these questions create conflicts that are nearly unresolvable. Health policy threatens to become captive to subjective fears. The boundlessness and undecidability of risk should warn us of the problems of preventive health.

Boundlessness of Risk Reduction

The basic conceptual problem is that there is no rational limit to risk reduction, no objective level of acceptable risk.[3] A risk can always be lower, so there is always an incentive to lower it, especially if focused only on a single risk factor. We see this in medical guidelines. Guidelines for healthy cholesterol have gotten progressively lower over the last few decades.[4] It seems that risks for cardiovascular events can always be reduced by reducing blood cholesterol levels, and thus experts even toy with setting target levels outside social or even species-normal levels.[5] There is always room to further minimize such risks. This tendency is not illogical, as reducing these levels actually does seem to reduce some risks of disease. Yet there is a danger to any goal that can become unlimited.

To see why, compare the logic of risk reduction to Aristotle's analysis of greed. As Aristotle notes, most natural desires are self-limiting: for example, the worst glutton will eventually be full.[6] The desire for money, however, is the desire for an abstraction, an abstract, quantifiable unit of exchange. There is no limit to it, because you can always have more money, so it stretches to infinity. The unbounded nature of the desire for money creates the problem of greed, an insatiable, destructive appetite.

Analogously, traditional forms of curative medical care are self-limiting. They reach their end once the disease is healed, suffering relieved, or function restored. There is a natural telos, even if it cannot always be reached. In contrast, risk, as a statistical description of the characteristics of a population, is a mathematical abstraction, similar to money. It too can proceed to infinity, although in this case it is the goal of making risk indefinitely small. The logic of risk aims at its elimination, which is what we see with these ever-reducing guidelines.

Yet the good life cannot aim at a limitless good because it is by definition unreachable. Seeking such a goal threatens to become all-consuming. Aristotle's critique of greed for money can be applied to unconstrained risk reduction for the sake of health: it leads one to be "serious about living, but not about living well."[7] One cannot flourish if the goods one pursues are unreachable in principle. The quest to reduce health risk soon runs into very pragmatic limits because of the side effects of risk reduction.

This theoretical momentum behind risk reduction is reinforced by all of the incentives in our society that push toward lowering the threshold of acceptable risk. In our safety-obsessed culture, no one will be blamed for extra precautions. Patient advocacy groups tend to always argue for more screening, more genetic testing, more treatment of risk. Even our models for producing knowledge skew toward increasing risk-reducing medication. Almost all clinical research trials, including those on risk reduction, are funded by pharmaceutical companies, whose bias would be toward greater consumption of risk-reducing medication.[8] There are problems with this research, but one need not impute fraud or sinister motives to researchers (and indeed much pharma research is of high quality) to note that there are conflicts of interest here that shape how research is performed and evaluated.[9] At the very least, our funding structure discourages certain kinds of studies: on the long-term consequences of being on a drug, on when it is acceptable to stop using a drug, and so on. These are the kinds of studies that would impede the momentum of risk reduction.

Breadth of Risk

Not only is there no natural limit to the minimization of risk, but also there is no conceptual framework for constraining the breadth of risks analyzed. A patient could be at risk for literally any condition. This is the danger revealed through the concrete problem of polypharmacy: patients taking many drugs to reduce risks of prediabetes, prehypertension, and other conditions at the same time. The problem is that as a patient consumes more medications, the risks of drug interactions, and thus side effects, grow. New technologies make this issue of breadth of risk much, much worse. Genetic risk analysis as developed in precision medicine, especially as it is used in conjunction with machine learning systems, takes this problem to a new extreme with the ability to indicate any number of hundreds of health risks.

For a concrete example of this problem, we can look to some of the proof-of-concept high-tech concierge care businesses that have arisen in the past decade, like the Pioneer 100 Wellness project discussed in the opening chapter. Or take Human Longevity Incorporated, founded by Craig Venter. It provides patients with whole-genome sequencing analyzed using the latest genomic information, comprehensive metabolomics, and a suite of other tests, including CT scans, echocardiography, and continuous cardiac monitoring.[10] These companies promise to give their patients a health edge through new technologies, especially genomic screening. What one actually finds is that almost everyone has some kind of predisease when examined this thoroughly. Human Longevity Incorporated found a number of undiagnosed genetic issues and previously undetectable metabolite abnormalities. All these findings lead to further surveillance. As you look for more risks, you find them. As more conditions are surveilled, more people will be found to be at risk. Even if one could find a way to constrain the perpetual minimization of risk, risk-based medicine would generate ever more patients, just because of the broadening scope of vision. Everyone is at risk for something; it is just a question of whether we want to live under a cloud of risk.

Thus the risk framework is dangerous because conceptually there is no way to constrain either its intensity or its breadth. The body is revealed to be ever more dangerous as new conditions are examined. Thinking in terms of risk brings its own momentum, a dynamic of expanded intervention, unless one takes concrete steps to limit it because of intellectual commitments beyond the risk paradigm. If risk-thinking is not self-limiting, and thus there is no neutral ground to constrain it, other ways must be sought to determine acceptable levels of risk and surveillance.

Political Concern with Health

The danger is not merely that concerns over risk will spread in the field of health. Rather, the true danger is that the management of health risk will take precedence over all other matters of public concern and all other ways of describing social problems. Taken as a right, it demands a political response. Health risk is a totalizing discourse that threatens to crowd out other ways of conceptualizing these problems. We no longer share a common moral language that can properly delineate different types of goods.[11] Thus political discourse is left with goals like income or health as the only things at which public policy can aim.[12] Among these, health is perhaps the only one that can gain universal approval. Therefore, medicalization becomes one of society's only grounds for justifying social intervention.

The lack of shared ends indicates the true importance of the language of social determinants of health. It allows policymakers to translate broader social problems and injustices into the shared language of health. Perhaps people cannot agree on a common language for justice that would indicate broad wealth inequalities as a moral failure, but public health can show that inequality raises risks for heart attacks. Perhaps we lack a language of human rights to describe the absence of clean water as a moral violation, but we can point to deaths caused by diarrheal disease as a metric to change. Thus health becomes a, perhaps the only, shared goal.

While seemingly a good end, a government's concern with its citizens' health can also take a dark turn tied to suspicions of degenerating health. Scholars have noted that the modern state's interests in the health of its citizens arise from reasons of state power.[13] It leads to beneficent state institutions, like national healthcare, but also has justified increased state control in dangerous ways. For example, eugenics arose out of fears over the future health of citizens and the implications for state power. Eugenics gained legislative force in the United States following results from IQ testing of World War I draftees showing lower levels of intelligence among certain groups.[14]

The foreword to a book on maintaining health from this era illustrates these fears over the citizen's health, with former President Taft describing how "the test of war . . . revealed the startling degree of physical insufficiency that characterizes civilized man all over the world. According to General Crowder's report, close to 35 per cent. of the men called in the draft were disqualified for active military service because of physical defects."[15] In the military struggle between states, the health of the population was critical: "At the foundation of national strength lies human vitality." Taft therefore saw it as an "urgent duty of all citizens to make themselves in the highest degree fit."[16] In this quote we see but one instance of the growing demand, a moral demand, for citizens to ensure their health for the common good. Taft cites a duty to ensure the highest degree of health, corresponding to the WHO's right to health. Eugenicists cited fears not only over military readiness but also over the ability of citizens to contribute to economic development or whether people would be a drain on the newly developing social insurance systems. This is just an extreme instance of the shared political language of health closely complementing the role of health in state interests, leading to government becoming a manager of health risks.[17]

The Failure of the Shared Language of Health Risk

Despite its prominence, minimizing risks to health is not a value upon which the common good can be built, because of the limitless nature of risk reduction. First, health risk now embraces a vast number of social activities. Yet risk management in any one of these domains raises other kinds of risks to life.[18] For example, environmental pollution reduces life expectancy, but it is unclear by how much because of the difficulty of the epidemiological research necessary to acquire that knowledge. Regulations that reduce pollution will lead some businesses to close, increasing certain kinds of unemployment and decreasing economic growth. These consequences will also affect health, especially of the laid-off workers, because of correlations between wealth, economic growth, and health. Yet these consequences are also difficult to quantify. The people protected by reduced pollution and those harmed by unemployment may very well be different groups. These conflicting interests set the stage for social struggle.

A similar problem was seen with Covid-19 lockdowns. Public health authorities assumed that Covid lockdowns would protect people from the spread of disease. They also knew that lockdowns would cause health decrements due to economic decline and the mental health effects of social isolation. These effects are hard to quantify, and they strike different social groups, with Covid striking older adults hardest and the effects of lockdowns disproportionately affecting workers and the young. Just as with individual management of health risk, social management of risk soon runs into undecidable questions regarding side effects. In the policy sphere, these issues set up unresolvable social conflicts.[19]

Conflicts over risk are not resolvable through cost/benefit analysis. First, the research is just too contested.[20] Epidemiology is notably uncertain and difficult, and the kinds of randomized controlled trials necessary are not possible, or at least affordable, for many of the questions we would like answered.[21] The research is even more challenging because most of it is undertaken by highly interested parties, creating threats of bias, and some parties even deliberately try to muddy the waters through the kinds of tactics engaged in by the tobacco industry.[22] Objective cost/benefit analysis becomes nearly impossible under these circumstances. Further, subjective values must be quantified, as in metrics like QALYs or DALYs, in which the value of a year of life with a disability or a disease must be compared against the value of an average year of healthy life.[23] Cost comparison is further complicated when other values, like natural beauty measured against a polluted environment, or the good of social interaction versus the health effects of lockdowns, must be integrated into the analysis. There is no objective way to balance the risks or costs.

Even if one were dealing with only one risk, there is the question of what is an acceptable level of risk to health. Risk can always be reduced, so there is always a more intensive intervention possible. How does one decide at what level to accept risk? This is not just a dispassionate, technocratic question. As the first chapter described, health risks are sensed not as future possibilities but as present assaults on well-being. To describe a person's risk as acceptable is to say that the disruption to their sense of being at home in their body is acceptable. It is experienced as a personal attack, and accepting another's being at risk seems unjust. One need only look to fierce debates among advocacy groups that occur when the U.S. Preventive

Services Task Force tries to change guidelines, like reducing the number of women subject to mammography,[24] to realize that these are not calm expert debates. Determining how much risk is acceptable makes a fundamental claim about values. The population phenomenon of risk becomes translated into personal fear of risks and personal feelings of injustice.

Given the lack of objective, rational grounds for prioritizing risks or deciding upon acceptable levels of risk, politics threatens to become a scramble of interest groups trying to control which risks are prioritized. The decisions on the control of risk become pure politics driven by interest groups and patient activists.[25] Any decision as to what would be acceptable risk is arbitrary, as there are no rational grounds for decision.[26] Preventive medicine, as it enters politics, will ultimately be a destabilizing force.

— Health risk will be an unstable ground both for individual medical decisions and for political negotiations of social issues. Yet in that very instability it creates the justification for the expansion of administrative procedures of control. Risk can always be reduced, but only at the price of greater intervention. Since risk reduction is now an aspect of social justice, the ground is laid for ever-greater medicalization. Risk reduction also becomes a moral demand, both for the state, which must ensure the right to health as articulated by the WHO, and for the individual. A healthy population is necessary for the common good, as Taft argues. The next chapters will describe the ethical problems with the expansion of this system of control and the related ethical demands.

SEVEN

Managing Populations

Many employees start the benefit year with an invitation to participate in a wellness program. These programs, which are sponsored by employers and insurance companies, try to decrease health spending by encouraging employees to engage in surveillance and consequent lifestyle coaching. The participants monitor their physiological risk factors like blood pressure or weight, commit to a program of exercise, or stop smoking. While much of what these programs do is beneficial, they may expand and intensify in troubling ways in the future. A section of one of the recent bills to replace the Affordable Care Act would even have allowed wellness programs to require genetic testing as part of participation.[1] Further, though generally voluntary, wellness programs can have a coercive edge. Currently these programs use the carrot of reduced health insurance premiums, up to 30 percent, to encourage participation. As health insurance premiums continue to rise, the carrot of reduced premiums could quickly become a stick of unaffordable premiums for those who refuse to engage with these programs or who are unresponsive to coaching. This paradigm would then be enforced by institutional sanction.

Workplace wellness programs demonstrate the features of preventive medicine identified in the first part of the book. Suspicion of people drives a need for surveillance. Their health behavior must be objectified and optimized. This management of people is driven by population-level analysis. This chapter examines the dynamics of this suspicion of the population body. The problems start with the fact that, as more and more risks are controlled by the modern state and its medical system, costs of healthcare rapidly rise. One response to increasing health costs is to ration care, but that is a deeply unpopular step. Instead, health policy has turned toward prevention with the idea that earlier treatment is cheaper. Yet some people are uncooperative; they just will not engage the prevention regime by stopping smoking, losing weight, or knowing their number. These patients threaten the financial viability of the system. Moreover, some medical practitioners also fail in the task of optimally managing risks through prescriptions and treatments. Public health managers must then step in to control these unruly actors and to make them better managers of risk, which, as we will see, threatens to undermine important human goods.

The Crisis of Cost in Healthcare

The introduction of Medicare and Medicaid led to a rapid expansion of medical infrastructure and the use of healthcare. The costs of the programs quickly exploded, so since the 1980s, health policymakers have sought ways to decrease medical costs. The first attempts at cost control sought to ration medical care. Insurance companies tried rationing by rejecting people who seemed as if they would cost too much. The sick, defined as people with preexisting conditions, were rejected from private health insurance as substandard risks. This strategy is a classic tool of insurance, but it clashed with changing understandings of justice. As the ability to control or insure against risk became an essential part of justice, the rejection of preexisting conditions came to be seen as fundamentally unjust insofar as the lack of insurance forced people to live with the risks of untreated illness and the resulting financial ruin. Thus the Affordable Care Act forced insurers to accept patients with preexisting conditions.

If health systems cannot ration insurance through the market, then another strategy is to ration care. Since much of the expense of healthcare is caused by costly drugs, surgeries, and other technological innovations, health systems could save money by refusing to pay for treatments that they do not deem cost-effective. In this schema, cost-effectiveness means that the cost of the treatment per life year saved falls below a certain agreed-upon value.[2] In general, attempts at cost containment principally address treatment for felt diseases. Cost-effectiveness analysis was tried by many entities, such as the U.K.'s National Institute for Health and Care Excellence (NICE), Oregon's Medicaid program, and Health Maintenance Organizations (HMOs), and much ink was spilled in bioethics in the 1990s in attempts to outline ethical modalities for rationing.[3]

Ultimately, this kind of explicit rationing of healthcare also proved unacceptable. Stories emerged of patients denied treatments, or of doctors wrestling with insurers. Under increasing public and political pressure, HMOs were unable to hold the line on rationing care. That is not to say that patients are not still denied treatments, that medications may not be on the formulary of a particular insurer, or that insurers might not make it difficult to gain approval for a treatment. Yet restrictions are nowhere near as great as HMOs had planned on or as would be necessary for true cost control. Almost all insurers cover procedures and devices approved by the Centers for Medicare and Medicaid Services (CMS), and CMS is statutorily required to approve treatments that are safe and effective.[4] When the idea of cost-effectiveness analysis emerged again in the first decade of this century, it was decried as the road to death panels. Thus explicit rationing has proven politically unpalatable.

With the failure of rationing and cost-effectiveness, attention has turned to prevention. The idea is that treating disease early will be cheaper than treating it later. Some scholars argue that prevention reduces costs, but economic analyses suggest that the large costs from a greater number of people on preventive regimens will outweigh savings from the few whose diseases would be prevented.[5] For example, cancer screening costs money because of the diagnostic imaging involved. If screening identifies new cancer patients, their treatment will cost money that otherwise might not be spent. Cancer survivors will use drugs to prevent recurrence and will be subject to increased levels of surveillance, meaning more costs.[6] To take another example, when guidelines for acceptable levels of blood pressure, cholesterol, or sugar levels are lowered, more people become at risk and are put on medication. Overdiagnosis is expensive, so surveillance and overtreatment add to medical costs. Moreover, even if a person saved the cost of treatment for a disease at a young age, that person will probably merely get another disease later in life that will require treatment, so prevention merely shifts costs onto Medicare. After all, the ultimate death rate is one per person.[7]

Even so, the early 2000s saw the embrace of health policy paradigms like population health or value-based care (VBC). VBC was developed by Donald Berwick and his colleagues to pursue what they called the Triple Aim: better health outcomes, better individual care experiences, and decreased cost.[8] Health systems could achieve this Triple Aim by pursuing quality and risk reduction. These goals would prevent costly errors and catch diseases before they became expensive, thus improving the health of the population.

Meeting the Triple Aim, though, required a single entity to assume responsibility for a particular population, an entity that Berwick called an integrator. The integrator could be a health system that provided most of the Medicaid care to a particular city; it could be an insurance company that covered many businesses in an area; it could be an HMO with a large presence in a city. Whatever form it took, the integrator had to be incentivized to advance the long-term health of a particular population rather than just make money off providing more and more surgeries, medications, and so on.

These incentives included reimbursements to providers tied to quality metrics:[9] Are people frequently readmitted to the hospital shortly after discharge, indicating poor planning for their release? Are there avoidable medical errors in the hospital? By addressing such problems, integrators could save large amounts of money while improving patient health, in theory. If the hospital improved these metrics, the integrator would increase its reimbursement rate, paying it a certain percentage in addition to the normal charge. If the hospital performed poorly on these measures, it would receive a penalty that would lower its payment by a certain percentage. Another tool for VBC is capitated payments. Under this framework, a health system is paid a set amount for each patient over the course of the year, no matter what health needs the patient might have. If patients are healthy, not needing much care, then the health system will profit. If patients are unhealthy, needing unplanned surgeries or hospital stays, then the health system will lose money. The health system's yearly profits are determined by the average cost of their patient population, so they are incentivized to keep patients healthy in a cost-effective manner.

To meet these incentives, integrators must exert more control. They have to ensure that doctors are providing high-quality care and that patients are complying with that care. They must determine that risks are sufficiently reduced. Exerting this control requires greater surveillance of workers and patients. Integrators must know what is happening in clinics and in patients' lives. It is for this reason that the implementation of electronic medical records (EMRs) was such a central feature of the Affordable Care Act. EMRs allow for much easier and more widespread surveillance of the medical workforce. Finally, for this control to be properly executed, health managers must be able to easily track and compare outcomes. For this tracking, they need quantitative metrics that allow for the surveillance and control of the medical workforce.

The Problems of Controlling Performance

This heavy development of performance metrics vastly expands the impact of risk reduction in medicine. To see why, let us first examine how risk reduction is pragmatically limited in the medical encounter. One obvious possible way to do so, dear to the bioethics community, is to let the patient determine the acceptable level of risk. This is the dream of autonomy; let the patient decide if she wants to get a mammogram or take statins. She can assess what level of risk she finds acceptable in her current life circumstances and proceed accordingly.

Yet foisting preventive health decisions on the individual is not tenable because people have a difficult time assessing risk and probability. In the last half century, behavioral economists have focused on the problems of "bias," really just difficulty with engaging certain kinds of statistical framing.[10] Thus autonomy alone is not the solution, because the patient must be educated on the risks and benefits of complex, probabilistic treatment regimes. Much progress has been made in how to appropriately format this kind of patient education about risk, but even the information supplied by better educational materials must be translated from the abstract level of the population into the concrete lived experience of the patient. For example, perhaps the elderly patient who lives alone is more fearful of the risks of a fall than the risks of high blood pressure, and thus it would be appropriate to let his blood pressure numbers rise. In the realm of diabetes treatment, Annemarie Mol describes the tinkering necessary to get a therapeutic regimen to fit with the habits and goals of a patient.[11] The medical practitioner plays a key role in this work of translation. Therefore, shared decision-making between the practitioner and patient is key for effective risk management.

Much of the effectiveness of this shared decision-making relies on the quality of a doctor's prudential judgment. Relying on both clinical experience and empathetic engagement with the patient's values, the practitioner must interpret abstract scientific facts about risk in terms of the patient's current life experience in order to achieve the patient's desired treatment goals. This sensitivity to the individual, concrete situation is what makes medicine an art rather than merely a scientific discipline. Classic descriptions of the healing relationship note the vital importance of this attention to specificity in clinical judgment.[12]

The language of precision medicine holds forth the promise of aiding a more personalized focus through individualized prediction of risk. As others have noted, though, risk prediction is not truly personalized.[13] Instead, it merely stratifies people into different risk groups, segmenting a population. Better than treating everyone the same, perhaps, but still not personalized. Moreover, these precision medicine readouts of risk analyze only those things that can be quantified. There is so much to clinical judgment that cannot be translated into metrics and that have a hard time finding a home in the prespecified boxes of an EMR: all the details of context within which the person lives, the themes that emerge from the narrative of her life history, and her values. The medical practitioner, however, can engage this rich picture of the patient through the engagement of prudence.

In so doing, the practitioner translates the information about risk for the patient by showing how the different options fit the patient's medical situation and treatment aims, and then makes a recommendation based on the patient's values and the practitioner's knowledge. This is not paternalistic because the practitioner is engaged in dialogue with the patient both pre- and post-judgment in order to ensure that the therapeutic regimen aims at the patient's good as the patient understands it. In any event, behavioral economics has shown that it is fanciful to think that practitioners can present information about risks in a way that would not sway the patient's decision. Framing effects, like the difference between explaining a treatment as giving a 40 percent chance of cure versus a 60 percent chance of death, are just too large, and there are good reasons for patients to attend to practitioners' framing. It is thus better to be conscious and intentional about how one frames the options.

Yet using the practitioner's prudential judgment to solve the problem of the logic of indefinite risk reduction is put in danger in the current institutional and economic organization of medicine. The reason is that risk management is envisioned not only as a way to improve health but also as a way to contain costs at the level of the population. Current models of health policy think in terms of populations, and thus the individual and context can be lost. Though VBC may speak of improving the experience of an individual patient, its concrete mechanisms of implementation belie that promise. To improve outcomes at reduced price, VBC bases reimbursement rates on metrics, ostensibly metrics that aim at maintaining health but in fact mean managing risk. For example, the quality metrics that govern reimbursement rates in VBC should be outcome metrics like number of deaths, heart attacks, and hospital readmissions, and many are.[14] However, it is difficult to equalize outcome metrics between different health systems because outcomes will in large part depend on the starting population. For example, a clinic in a poor inner-city area with a heavy burden of chronic disease, homelessness, and drug use will nearly always have worse outcomes than a clinic in a wealthy suburb for reasons beyond the quality of care given in the clinic. Because of this, many quality metrics often are what are called process metrics:[15] Are statins prescribed when risk of heart attack rises to a certain level? Is metformin prescribed when there is some percentage risk of diabetes? Many of these process metrics relate to managing risk.

This management of population risk thus affects clinical judgment. For example, the surgeon George Sarosi tells the story of an elderly patient who arrived at his yearly checkup with relatively high cholesterol levels and elevated blood sugar.[16] Though the man had no observable pathologies, these elevated numbers indicated a future risk of disease. Because his clinic focused on high-value care through following guidelines, his doctors sought to control his blood pressure and blood sugar by using increasingly powerful medications at higher doses. Under this intensive treatment regimen, the patient began to feel light-headed when he stood up and frequently awoke in the middle of the night needing to go to the bathroom. Eventually, he fell during one of these nighttime trips to the bathroom because of a dangerously low blood pressure, breaking his hip in the process. The surgery to repair the hip did not go well, leading to postoperative complications, and the patient will never live independently again. Moreover, he has been nearly bankrupted by medical bills. As Sarosi puts it, "His doctor may have received a bonus for adhering to the guidelines, but Mr. O lost his home and independence." This anecdote illustrates a broader problem with VBC: the practitioner is no longer considering only whether this risk-reducing pharmaceutical is right for this patient given his total life and medical circumstances. She is also considering how the decision to prescribe or, especially, not to prescribe this medication will affect her quality metrics and thus reimbursement scores.[17] This is the whole point of incentive systems, to shift practitioners' judgment to consider the desired metrics. Predictive risk is meant to play an ever-larger role in the practitioner's judgment. Thus these current systems of risk management cannot but disrupt the prudential judgment of the practitioner, forcing her to attend to the external goods of institutional reimbursement rather than just the internal goods of the healing relationship. This loss of clinical judgment is important because the tools of medicine can be dangerous and good practitioners know that their first imperative is to not harm the patient through their action.

These trends will be accelerated as different kinds of information and tools are integrated into the clinical workflow, such as machine learning–driven clinical decision support systems or the inclusion of genetic information in EMRs. AI-driven clinical decision support systems will result from the analysis of the vast amounts of data provided by precision medicine programs. In this kind of planned automated system, messages will pop up during a clinical encounter suggesting that the practitioner prescribe something or perform some test. They continually will inform the doctor how to reduce risk in line with health systems' priorities. Genetics and machine learning will predict more forms of risk than straightforward guidelines as they plumb ever-larger datasets to find all the patient's risks. The promised automation of risk prediction and the integration of machine learning systems in the clinic raise deep problems for clinical judgment. Automating decisions on prescriptions of risk-reducing medications raises three problems: those of explainability, liability, and disposition.

First, if the practitioner believes a prescription is not called for in the face of the system's recommendation, she must determine the grounds for rejecting that recommendation. In the case of a clinical guideline, a doctor can at least point to the studies and evidence used in justifying it and say that this patient does not fit the criteria of the body of evidence that led to the guideline for some reason. AI systems cannot be challenged in the same way. Usually, one does not know the particular reasons as to why the system made a particular prediction. Machine learning systems are designed to pick out patterns humans cannot recognize. These programs are black boxes, neither explainable nor transparent, and that is what makes them so effective.[18] Thus there is no ground for argument with them because the user does not understand them. This feature of these systems compounds a further problem in that clinicians generally do not have the expertise to appraise genetic information. Without the possibility of engaging in reasoned argumentation, there is no space for prudential judgment. We are left with a battle of authorities: the practitioner's versus the machine's.

It is not at all clear that the human will win in this clash of authorities. These systems are implemented by managers exactly because of a distrust of and desire to control the human factor. While practitioners certainly make many mistakes, so do guidelines and computer systems, especially once they emerge from the idealized world of clinical trials into the messy world of everyday clinical practice. Still, one of the major concerns in clinical ethics is over whether practitioners will be able to reject these machine judgments without facing the threat of greater liability.[19] If the practitioner rejects the machine's recommendation and the patient suffers an adverse outcome, as some will in any case, the practitioner will be open to greater scrutiny and lawsuits. Even if practitioners are not concerned about malpractice lawsuits from patients, they will be concerned about reductions to their reimbursement rates by management. In the face of such threats from management and courts, they will likely become ever more amenable to just acquiescing to what the system suggests.

Third, increased acquiescence to these systems does not even have to feel like a conflict. Studies of human-technology interaction describe the phenomenon of automation bias. This is when users become more and more trusting of automated systems the more they use them. Their senses and intuitions become dulled to the point of following the system's directives in the face of overwhelming counterevidence.[20] Practitioners become deskilled, losing the ability to make their own judgments. The best examples of deskilling and automation bias occur among pilots, with many examples of plane crashes caused by pilots becoming disoriented or unable to reassert control in an unusual situation because of their overreliance on automated control systems. In the medical case, this would mean trusting risk prediction in the face of polypharmacy or life circumstances that make it unwise. Automated risk management will detract from practitioners' capacity for prudential judgment, increasingly making them merely a component of the machine.[21]

Even those most committed to VBC as an ideal are recognizing the problem with management through metrics. As Donald Berwick, the architect of VBC, describes, "Measurement in health care has gone wild."[22] Bureaucracies are too demanding, overwhelming practitioners with requests for data. Many of these metrics are not very informative. Placed in the perspective of the dangers of a focus on risk, even somewhat informative metrics can cause harm. There is thus an urgent need to rein in this apparatus of surveillance and control.

Suspicions of the Other

The most intense pressure is exerted on doctors at the moment, but it is spreading to patients. In the wellness programs described in the opening to this chapter, insurers and corporations use financial incentives to surveil employee health metrics and affect their health behaviors. VBC providers have specialized programs for high-risk groups that involve more intensive engagement with a greater focus on social services, as well as more surveillance.[23] It is thus not only doctors that need to be managed for VBC to work.

Because of large government spending on healthcare, broader public policy tools are being brought to bear on population risks. Take, for instance, the debates surrounding taxes or bans on large sodas. Because obesity is a major risk factor for many diseases, health policy experts want to lower the average weight of the population, lowering levels of obesity. One source of excess calories in the U.S. diet is high-sugar sodas. Higher taxes on these would incentivize people to drink less, much as high taxes on cigarettes decrease smoking. For these reasons, New York City introduced a ban on sugary drinks in 2012. The tax led to an outcry about state control over consumer choice and was soon overturned by court challenges.[24] However, it is merely an extension of the logic of population-level risk reduction that requires using as many policy levers as possible to shape outcomes.

While the limitation of prudence required by these efforts at incentivization and nudging raises ethical questions,[25] a deeper concern regards the more intensive focus of state power on health risks. Already with Covid we saw the imposition of nearly total control on society to manage infectious disease risk.[26] We are also seeing this expansion of control, albeit less extreme, with regard to other health risks. The danger is that, as in the case in the doctor's office, much will be missed by the technocratic gaze of the public health specialist. Just as public health officials ignored threats to children's education, to mental health, or to substance abuse caused by pandemic risk control measures, they will probably miss other dangers of risk reduction in relation to noninfectious diseases. Moreover, as risk remains recalcitrant, since it will never decrease to zero, policymakers are forced to use ever more intrusive measures to bring risks under control. At its logical extreme, as in the pandemic, it undermines systems of checks and balances. Policymakers thus try to foster a moral obligation to minimize health risk, the topic of the next chapter.

EIGHT

The Obligation of Health

Precision and preventive medicine gain their moral force from the general recognition that health is a good. Because it is a good, people are under some kind of imperative or moral obligation to preserve health.[1] Though not everyone would frame this obligation in the same way, there are shared moral intuitions about the value of pursuing health. For example, economists assume that health is a good that libertarian paternalism can validly promote.[2] Or disagreement over whether the terminally ill can take their life should not obscure the broad support for suicide prevention programs.[3] Further, bioethicists may uphold autonomy in medical decision-making as a fundamental principle of medical ethics, yet few medical practitioners or ethicists are willing to countenance without challenge a seemingly irrational rejection of a nonburdensome life-saving treatment with a high chance of success. Health as a good demands some sort of care.

The obligation to preserve health can be defended in several ways. Some scholars take a natural law or Aristotelian approach: health is a basic, natural good for the kind of creatures humans are, so we should seek it as a part of our natural end.[4] For others, health might be merely a rational desire, since health is necessary for pursuing other goods and projects. Beyond its value for the individual, health is also a social good. It allows us to better serve the common good, so we are under some sort of social obligation to preserve our lives in the interests of family, nation, and other groups in which we participate. For many religions, life is a gift from God that we must treat with respect. There are thus many reasons to see preserving health as some sort of duty.

Traditionally, though, the obligation to preserve health and life was fairly limited. It enjoined the person to procure the basic necessities of food, shelter, and clothing; to not commit suicide; and to seek basic, widely available medical care. Note that this last aspect regarded felt illness; it was a duty to respond to the disharmony in one's body. Once the definition of health changes to embrace risk reduction, however, the understanding of the duty to preserve health also changes. Preserving health now means minimizing risk. It is no longer sufficient for the person to avoid starving or killing himself. Instead, risk-reducing interventions are necessary. Through this shift, the duty to preserve health threatens to become an unlimited task, not only on the level of the state, as chapter 6 described, but also for the individual.

This chapter examines how the understanding of the individual obligation to preserve health is shifting as preventive medicine gains force. Debates within the Roman Catholic tradition of casuistry surrounding the duty to pursue medical treatment serve to illustrate the new nature of the obligation. Catholic casuistry is one of the most well-developed discourses on this obligation,[5] but, in recent years some Catholic bioethicists have begun arguing for an expanded understanding of this obligation based on ideas of healthcare as risk reduction. Though secular bioethics gives less explicit direction on these obligations, these expanded duties also appear in secular programs and discourses. The end of this chapter will show that these shifts are not limited to religious ethics but reflect broader developments in secular society.

Expanding Obligations to Health

The obligation to maintain health in the Catholic tradition is implied by the commandment not to kill.[6] The commandment enjoins each person to have a reverence for life, which goes beyond a mere prohibition of killing to become a duty to care for the life of both others and oneself.[7] This commitment to care for the sick led to early Christian efforts in healthcare, such as the first hospitals and ambulance services.[8] While late antique and medieval theologians touched on these duties, it was early modern scholastics who developed an extensive casuistry surrounding what kinds of treatments a Christian is obligated to pursue. Drawing from a casuistry on food and medical care that begins with the Spanish Dominican theologian Francisco de Vitoria in the sixteenth century, ordinary means of preserving life came to be defined as those kinds of means that a person was obligated to use, whereas extraordinary means were not obligatory, although they could still be used.[9]

In this tradition, the obligation to preserve life is a limited one for at least two reasons. First, there are other goods that are more important than life. For example, one can sacrifice one's life out of love for others, commitment to truth, or protection of the common good. A person can even risk his health because of a commitment to a penitential form of life.[10] Spiritual care comes before physical. Thus the good of health is a subordinate good.

Second, because it seeks a good, preserving life is not an absolutely binding duty.[11] Absolutely binding duties are those things that must always be done. Usually, such perfect duties refer to negative commandments, like do not kill the innocent or do not steal, which are absolutely binding. People can always avoid violating these duties by just avoiding the forbidden action, even if it entails danger to themselves. In contrast, positive commandments prescribe actions that seek goods, such as giving alms. A person should frequently give alms, and giving alms is good for both her own virtue and the recipient's material well-being, but the person does not have to spend all her time giving alms; there are other duties to which she must attend. An individual occasion for alms-giving becomes an absolute duty only in pressing need. More generally, there are multiple goods that we could pursue and realize at any moment: caring for our children, seeking knowledge, promoting health, or performing acts of charity. All of these are duties in some way, but they cannot all be done at the same time. Each person must prioritize which goods to pursue on the basis of her own situation, vocation, and prudence. Positive duties can be forgone for a proportionate reason.

Thus, while the preservation of health is a good and something one should attend to, the *obligation* to actively preserve health is relatively limited. Ordinary care generally entails basic food, clothing, and medical care for present illness. No form of treatment is required if it is unduly burdensome because of pain, cost, inconvenience, and so forth. The judgment of these burdens, the relative chance of success of treatment, and thus the obligation to pursue treatment are always left to the prudential judgment of the individual patient.[12]

This quite limited obligation is also almost always discussed in the tradition in relation to a felt disease rather than future disease. The tradition merely requires that one not embark on a form of life or diet that is manifestly self-destructive. Yet even here, a person can pursue an asceticism that certainly will not maximize his life span, as long as it is an institutionally recognized practice rather than a personal eccentricity. There is very little discussion of preventive measures in the tradition. In fact, the sixteenth-century Jesuit Tomas Sanchez says that "one is not obliged to use medicines to prolong life even where there would be the probable danger of death, such as taking a drug for many years to avoid fevers, etc."[13] Such a viewpoint would certainly rule out statins as a moral obligation. Sanchez still asserts that "one is held however, while sick, to consult doctors and use what is healthful." He can make this distinction because he separates the duties regarding prevention from those regarding felt disease. Similarly, a recent statement by the Catholic Church's doctrinal body, the Congregation for the Doctrine of the Faith, said, "Vaccination is not, as a rule, a moral obligation."[14] There is no moral obligation to quit smoking or avoid obesity in order to preserve health. There may be other reasons that such actions can become obligations, such as the common good, the virtue of temperance, or the prevention of luxury, but health is not one of them. There are too many other considerations, too many goods to pursue, to make preventive health a moral obligation. Otherwise, life could become a maze of legalistic demands.

Orthodox Judaism provides a similar analysis. There too an extensive casuistry calls individuals to preserve their own and others' lives. Yet there is no obligation to seek screening tests.[15] The focus is on responding to felt disease: "Since the building blocks of the rabbinic vocabulary on ill health speak of 'discomfort' and 'inability to stand up,' the notion of illness simmering beneath a perception of well-being is alien to the rabbinic mentality."[16] There is no need to seek out ill health, especially as this search might introduce its own discomforts through anxiety.

Yet one can ask whether the obligations surrounding health change when society's understanding of health changes. If health is not merely the absence of disease, as it was when this distinction was developed, but the minimization of risk, then there may be much more that one must do to preserve health. If risk itself becomes disease, then treating risks becomes an obligatory form of care. The sphere of obligation then would become much broader. This expansion of the obligation to seek medical care is already under way among some Catholic bioethicists. Its roots lie in the embrace of risk as disease. Some textbooks in theological bioethics already define the risk of cancer as the presence of cancer.[17] Other bioethicists even allow for the use of biotechnological enhancements to pursue risk reduction in terms of cardiovascular function and bone density.[18] If health is a basic good, it can be sought as far as possible so long as one does not oppose another good. The Dominican bioethicist Nicanor Austriaco argues in favor of a genetic therapy that would eliminate the function of the *PCSK9* gene, which would lower "lipid levels below our species norms in order to decrease cardiovascular risk."[19] Here risk reduction as health promotion is added to medicine's more classic role of curing illness because "medicine seeks not only to restore, but to preserve and protect the health of individuals."[20] In this reading, it is licit to make people "healthier than healthy" through risk reduction because it aims at a human good. Though these authors would clearly not place health as the highest good, their arguments license a great expansion of risk reduction therapies. As Austriaco notes, "There is no straightforward response" to the question of how low LDL levels should be, implying that lower is almost always better.[21] Moreover, this argument opens up a vista of vastly expanded genetic interventions to lower risks of cancer, HIV, and other diseases.[22]

If risk is disease and any form of risk reduction is therapy, could it become an obligation? It seems so given the number of moral theologians willing to declare that receiving Covid-19 vaccinations is a moral obligation.[23] To be clear, I publicly and privately supported and encouraged Covid-19 vaccination as an effective means of addressing the dangers of the pandemic.[24] I even think there is an argument to be made for an obligation to receive common childhood vaccinations like MMR based on reasons of the common good rather than arguments that they are ordinary care.[25] Covid vaccines are different from these childhood vaccines in that one can still transmit the Covid virus after the vaccination and the vaccines have a much shorter window for reducing symptomatic infection (though they reduce risk of hospitalization and death for much longer). Whereas measles or polio vaccination drives give a good chance of eradicating these diseases, that is not the case with Covid vaccines. The person is merely, for a time, mildly affecting transmission dynamics. A valuable contribution, perhaps, but not the ground for a moral obligation, meaning that vaccine mandates are problematic.[26] The biggest effect is on personal health, making ordinary means of care the thing to argue over.

The argument that Covid vaccination is part of ordinary means of care proceeds, for these ethicists, from a citation of Thomas Aquinas's commentary on 2 Thessalonians: "It is prescribed that a human being sustains his body, for otherwise he murders himself.... Therefore, one is bound to nourish his body, and we are bound likewise with respect to all other things without which the body cannot live."[27] Recent authors then draw the implication that because we are obliged to eat, there is a moral obligation to preserve health. Vaccines preserve health. Ergo, there is a moral obligation to receive a vaccine.

There are clear problems with this line of argumentation. First, there is no recognition of the important difference between eating and vaccination to our survival. If I do not eat, I will surely die.[28] If I do not receive a vaccination, however, I merely increase my risk for death. Moreover, there are great differences in the relative risk between different age groups and health statuses.[29] Implicitly, these authors have equated risk reduction with eating, but these actions have a very different relationship to my continued existence.

For these authors, preserving life now means reducing risk. The implications of this argumentative strategy are vast, especially since the authors pay no attention to relative risks. Any risk reduction, be it pharmaceutical, surgical, or screening, would be, not merely a possibility to prudently reflect on, but a moral obligation that must be pursued. Perhaps there is some limitation they would put on risk reduction, but it is not in their writing.

Instead, the move to the vision of health as minimal risk has vastly expanded the sphere of medical obligation. If their analysis is correct, the Catholic now has an unbounded task of reducing risk, and the imperfect duty becomes a perfect, absolute imperative. However, the traditional analysis of these topics should warn us off this approach. Our interest in health is limited because of the many other goods that we can pursue. Of course, there are some risks that an individual should perhaps avoid because of being at particularly high risk or because of specific aspects of his vocation. Determining proper concern over risk is the task of prudence, though. A general obligation should apply only to basic needs for sustaining life and some treatments for serious, present illness.

Secular Imperatives

It may come as little surprise that religious traditions would embrace such obligations, but these obligations also exist in secular sources. After all, "Know your numbers" is just as much an imperative statement as "Pursue ordinary care." It is just less logically tenable, as we do not know how it receives its binding force.[30] Instead of clear arguments and the sanction of a tradition of reflection, individuals adopt normative demands for health through their interaction with institutions. These demands seem to arise from one's own desires but are frequently adopted as part of a much broader social formation.[31] Health has been proposed as one of our highest goods, and social forces drive us to pursue it at significant cost.

Thus wellness programs not only provide incentives and surveillance to help people achieve the goal of health. They also serve to educate people as to what kinds of goals they should pursue and what means they should use to pursue these goals. If these goals are not pursued, then coercive strategies like higher premiums can be applied. The ideal outcome, though, is for people to internalize these goals, to personally make health one of their highest goods.[32] Then individuals will pursue fitness and physiological surveillance without the need for structures and programs to enforce these norms. People, at least of a certain class, will pursue maximal physical ability, seeing it as equal to health.

There are three dangers to this approach. First, the imperative of health increases anxiety. The unhealthy person suffers not only from the illness itself but also from a feeling of moral and normative failure. Not only future illness is brought into the present but also future stigma. People will do much to escape this social stigma,[33] so the anxiety drives people to preserve health. Yet there is no way to relieve anxiety by satisfying this imperative. It is endless because there is always risk. There is always something more to do, a physiological marker to be optimized, a genetic risk to be neutralized. There is always surveillance and screening to endure. Even if one does all this, the person is still doomed to death. Death and ill health come for us all.

Second, intensified attention to health distracts us from pursuing other goods. There are only so many goods that we can pursue given our finite existence. Seeking reduced health risk means not pursuing other goods. Plato explored this danger in the *Republic*, in which he criticizes the rich man who spends his life focused solely on his health regimen rather than on the tasks necessary for the pursuit of the common good.[34] Today, as well, Barbara Ehrenreich describes the intensive health regimens of the world's affluent classes for whom "health is indistinguishable from virtue."[35] When health becomes the locus of virtuous activity, other pursuits, like service, fall by the wayside.

Third, the obligation to maximize health also causes people to deny the value of lives that have no chance of maximizing health and productivity, as demonstrated in attempts to prevent the birth of children with disabilities. Testing for congenital abnormalities during pregnancy is no longer really a choice to be made. It is the default option, almost a duty. Such tests are ordered along with all the other blood tests that monitor maternal health and risks to the child. Parents need to be aware of and consciously refuse such tests if they do not want the information so that they can avoid the eugenic temptation and pressure to judge a life with disability as less valuable and thus to destroy it. If they do not have these tests, they are violating one of our society's strongest imperatives of maximizing health. It is expressed, not on a list of "Thou shalts," but instead in the mundane procedures and regulations of healthcare and workplace insurance programs. Through these channels, along with media and other influences, the imperative of health becomes embedded to destructive effect. The next chapter will discuss this process in more depth.

NINE

Exclusion and Elimination

There are two different general strategies by which to control the risk of disease in a population. One approach tries to change the structure of the population as a whole,[1] by, for example, decreasing the average weight of the entire society or decreasing the average blood pressure of everyone. Most of preventive medicine tries to affect everyone's health, with interventions attempting to shift the entire normal curve of society. A second approach addresses only those at highest risk:[2] give statins only to people with the top 10 percent of blood cholesterol levels or at the highest risk for a cardiac event. Or concentrate lifestyle interventions on the morbidly obese. Instead of shifting the risk curve as a whole, such policies attempt only to eliminate the danger to the few people on the far right of the curve. The shift resulting from the intervention still affects population averages.

There is much to be said for this latter strategy, even it may not maximize the number of lives saved, and I will return to it in the last section of the book. It achieves the most cost-effective use of risk-reducing pharmaceuticals and screening programs by concentrating them on those at highest risk, which reduces the number needed to treat (NNT). It also leaves most of the population alone, not sweeping them into the ongoing cycle of preventive services, with all of their possible negative effects. Targeting those at high risk also gives the greatest attention to those who are in the most danger, who are frequently among the marginalized of society.[3]

To give two examples of such focused attention on the poor, first, directly observed therapy programs serve patients most at risk of not taking medications for HIV or tuberculosis.[4] The primary intervention involves health workers visiting patients every day to ensure that they take their medications. In the best cases, these visits build a system of social support for the patient. Since the risk of noncompliance (meaning not taking a prescribed medication) is frequently tied to social circumstances, such as poverty or substance use, many of these programs also provide case managers who connect patients to available social services. Similarly, many population health programs give special attention to high-risk patients,[5] such as patients with multiple diseases and complex socioeconomic circumstances, like homelessness or mental illness. These high-risk patients are assigned to complex care management programs, which address their medical issues through coordinated care and their social problems by connecting them to social welfare programs. Thus focusing on those at highest risk can embody a strategy of care that alleviates the effects of structural injustice.

There is another way to address the highest-risk patients, though. Instead of removing their risks through therapeutic engagement, one could simply remove them from the population, basically slicing off the right extreme of the bell curve of risk. Insurance companies do this when they refuse to cover preexisting conditions. They exclude high-risk individuals from their population. Even the high-risk patient programs described in the last paragraph illustrate the exclusion of the worst risks. Their care is not for the highest-risk patients as such; they care for the highest-risk patients whose costs of care can be reduced.[6] Therefore, they are constantly evaluating the patients in the program to determine whose involvement is proving cost-effective (i.e., which ones are responding, who is taking responsibility for themselves, who is reducing their need for care). Some patients will never transition out of their high-cost, high-risk status because of either their social circumstances or the nature of their disease. Patients who do not provide a return on investment are often cut from these programs. This selection for care among those at high risk demonstrates a more general feature of risk reduction: it tends to exclude or eliminate portions of the population whose risk cannot be controlled.[7] The current chapter explores the negative effects of this eliminative dynamic.

The Exclusion of the Risky

The program of indefinitely reducing risk raises a fundamental problem: What happens when it encounters those whose risks cannot be reduced? What happens to the people whose genetic diseases are almost certain to occur? What about patients whose genetic risk scores suggest a suite of possible problems that are not cost-effective to treat or that do not have risk-reducing treatments, such as Alzheimer's? What should we do with people who are consistently noncompliant with risk-reducing measures and thus run up extremely high costs? The only answer, it would seem, would be either to just accept those risks and costs or to exclude these high-risk patients from the population of interest. Since the former solution fails to follow the basic dynamic of risk reduction, policymakers are tempted toward exclusion.[8]

Let me give three examples of how this exclusion occurs. As noted above, the first and most obvious example occurs in insurance markets. Life or health insurers simply will not cover certain people. They are just at too great a risk of immediate death or expensive medical care. That is why life insurance classically demanded a medical examination and information about lifestyle.[9] It is why medical insurers excluded people with preexisting conditions. These people are not good risks in which to invest, so they are excluded.

Of course, exclusion from insurance causes immense suffering for those bankrupted by medical bills or families who lost a breadwinner with no life insurance to support them. Such suffering helped to encourage the development of social insurance systems from which no one would be excluded.[10] In turn, expanded eligibility for social insurance led to increased costs because the system was committed to cover those whose coverage was not cost-effective. Fears over the solvency and expanding costs of social support systems in part drove the eugenics movement. Eugenicists saw a future of ever-increasing demands on state care as the population became less and less fit, as more people with higher risks survived. By the telling of eugenicists, hereditary risk factors would only spread through the population, thereby swelling the ranks of those at high risk. They saw it as crucial to intervene early by sterilizing those who would give birth to the future high-risk individuals, eliminating these future people from the population.[11]

Though few people today would embrace the moniker of eugenics and even fewer would find state coercion acceptable for these goals, the basic strategy of eliminating the high-risk people of the future continues today. Genomic Prediction offers its PRSs so that parents can exclude the riskiest embryos from existence. Some bioethicists applaud a procreative beneficence that would use genetic screening technologies to select the child with the most chance of success, which generally means eliminating the children with the highest risk of ill health.[12] The eugenic risk paradigm is alive and well, though in a liberal form.

Finally, this eliminative threat also appears in the literature of population health. Thomas McKeown was a doctor who, more than anyone else, showed that the broad increase in life expectancy over the last two centuries was due to social determinants like food supply rather than anything done by medicine or even public health.[13] He noted that there were limits to what public health and social policy could achieve, though. At some point, population health would need to turn to genetic factors to deal with those conditions that were intractable to its other methods. Therefore, he thought "there are few more important tasks for medical research than the study of methods of recognizing abnormal embryos or foetuses early in pregnancy" for abortion.[14] This approach would be the only way to limit genetic disabilities and diseases. Population health is constantly tempted to turn to an eliminative paradigm. Its tools were developed by eugenicists, and its goals imply the ongoing reduction of risk. Eventually some people will stand in the way of risk reduction because of their constitution, social circumstances, or obstinate will.[15] The demand for control and the goal of indefinite risk reduction threaten their violent exclusion.

Fears for the Population's Future

Most of the analysis in this chapter addresses the problem of engaging people through population concepts. The inspiration to eliminate and exclude those at high risk emerges when they are viewed abstractly rather than seen in the fullness of their individuality. Yet the problem of anticipation, of bringing future ill health into the present, which I described in the first chapter as part of prevention, also appears here. The goal of hereditary risk reduction is to prevent disease in a future generation, to head off the cost, suffering, and death from illness. But in excluding or eliminating those at high risk, suffering and death are made present through forced sterilization, abortion, and the experience of exclusion.[16] It makes future disruption present in order to avoid what it thinks are worse possible future problems.

I am not arguing that elimination and exclusion are necessary or inevitable aspects of risk reduction programs. That would be foolish and countered by much historical evidence. Yet they are dangers created by the drive to optimize risks. If the tendency to indefinitely reduce risks is not countered by other influences, then it drifts toward these malicious results. Thankfully, risk reduction programs are generally inspired by a multitude of other goals and are run by people with broader ethical frameworks. The eliminative paradigm has historically been disturbingly common, though.

A proponent of risk reduction might protest this description. She might argue that the primary motivation for these programs of risk reduction is not exclusion. Instead, they are inspired by and aim at solidarity. The programs claim to seek the common good through their population measures. The next chapter will describe the ways in which such a claim is true, but also how risk reduction betrays older models of solidarity and community.

TEN

Caring for the Statistical Other

Perhaps the first written Christian engagement with epidemic disease was Cyprian of Carthage's *Mortality*. Beginning in approximately AD 250, a plague ravaged the Mediterranean world, lasting for the next fifteen years.[1] This Cyprianic Plague had a high death rate, reportedly killing five thousand people in one day in the city of Rome. In response to this crisis, Cyprian, as bishop of Carthage, took to the pulpit to preach to his frightened flock. He began with a description of the suffering caused by the disease: "That now the bowels loosened into a flux exhaust the strength of the body, that a fever contracted in the very marrow of the bones breaks out into ulcers of the throat, that the intestines are shaken by continual vomiting, that the blood-shot eyes burn, that the feet of some . . . are cut away by the infection of diseased putrefaction."[2] Then he proceeds to describe how his flock should interpret these sufferings: "All this contributes to the proof of faith. What greatness of soul it is to fight with the powers of mind unshaken against so many attacks of devastation and death, what sublimity to stand erect amidst the ruins of the human race . . . and to rejoice rather and embrace the gift of the occasion, which, while we are firmly expressing our faith, and having endured sufferings, are advancing to Christ by the narrow way of Christ."[3] If one can look beyond the elevated rhetoric of the trained lawyer, influenced as Cyprian was by the even more exaggerated style of Tertullian, one hears an important lesson: Cyprian is calling the Christians of Carthage to tame their fears.

A superficial reading could interpret this sentiment as naïve optimism, a belief that all will turn out fine and one need not worry about disease. But it is not. It is an outlook that accepts danger, even the danger of death, believing, with Pope Francis in the face of another pandemic, that God turns "to the good everything that happens to us, even the bad things."[4] Further, Cyprian did not think developing the courage to confront disease would be easy. This difficulty may account for the rhetorical fervor of his statements. He says that "these are trying exercises for us."[5] One must work to overcome fear, especially in the face of calamities. However, ultimately, nothing can separate a person from Christ's love.

Would this lack of fear not make people careless, even suicidal? No, because one of the reasons that Cyprian as well as other ancient philosophical sources like the Stoics wanted people to overcome their natural fear of death was so that they could better serve others.[6] Fear leads people to flee their duties when they may be dangerous or to turn away from an act of love that may bear risk. Cyprian's biographer describes such a situation during the outbreak: "All were shuddering, fleeing, shunning the contagion, impiously exposing their own friends, as if with the exclusion of the person who was sure to die of the plague, one could exclude death itself also.... No one did to another what he himself wished to experience."[7] Cyprian confronted this neglect of care, urging "the benefits of mercy," even for the non-Christians who had recently been their persecutors. He describes the disease not only as a test of faith but as a test of justice and charity: "whether the well care for the sick, whether relatives dutifully love their kinsmen as they should, whether masters show compassion to their ailing slaves, whether physicians do not desert the afflicted begging their help, whether the violent repress their violence, whether the greedy, even through the fear of death, quench the ever insatiable fire of their raging avarice, ... whether the rich, even when their dear ones are perishing and they are about to die without heirs, bestow and give something!"[8] Note that in each of these cases he calls for concrete care of others. Other historical sources describe the early church's active care for the sick through organized services such as stretcher-bearers.[9] These Christian responses to illness were remarked upon by non-Christians.[10]

To review, Cyprian calls for a twofold response to epidemics. First, on the personal, subjective side, one must avoid the fear and anxiety that presses down upon the person in such emergencies. Christians must hold fast to faith in the love and care of God. This faith gives a person the confidence to care for others despite risk, which is the second aspect of this response. By banishing anxiety, one has the courage to embrace charity for others by concretely meeting their needs, thus responding to God's love.[11] Absence of fear and active, direct care should thus characterize responses to pandemics.

I do not think that it is too controversial to say that very powerful forces push against this twofold stance. Instead of absence of fear, there is an epidemic of anxiety. Much of our media and government messaging directs our attention toward dangerous futures. Moreover, the response to the Covid-19 pandemic made direct care of others difficult. Of course, medical staff and other kinds of professionals provided direct care as part of their professional duties. But for the nonprofessional, many of the most obvious paths of direct care for others were blocked. Even visiting the sick for accompaniment or in order to offer the sacraments was disrupted. Older adults spent months in isolation. Alzheimer's patients and children with disabilities languished from lack of human contact. Data suggest that anxiety, depression, and drug use spiked. Compare Cyprian's recommendations for relating to families to public health advice. Cyprian calls people to "dutifully love their kinsmen as they should." In contrast, public health authorities recommended isolating the infected, even children insofar as possible, from the rest of the household for ten days.

In our current approach to pandemics and risk more generally, other individuals have become a threat. Instead of engaging concrete others, what we are called to do is to care for the population as a whole by attending to the shifting probabilities of disease and mortalities that our actions affect. Under the regime of risk, people still care, but that care is addressed to the statistical other, since the person will never know those whom his changed action, his social distancing may affect. The concrete other, far from being a target of care, becomes a source of danger. The concrete other must be avoided. We stand together by standing apart.

Solidarity and the Common Good

This example illustrates the paradox of another claim of preventive and precision medicine. On the one hand, preventive medicine enthusiasts see its various instantiations, like precision medicine, as ways to reinforce social solidarity. By caring for all of the population, precision medicine can become "We-medicine," as opposed to the "Me-medicine" of curative care or highly individualized prevention.[12] Population health turns toward the community and the common good, according to many bioethicists. In precision medicine, however, solidarity is not formed as a bond with concrete others or an actual community. Instead, it is solidarity with statistical others in a population. The common good is embodied in the statistical metrics of the population. However, by turning from the concrete other with whom one pursues a common end to the abstract population, these authors betray the original meaning of solidarity and the common good, or at least that is what this chapter argues.

In donning the mantle of solidarity, preventive medicine tries to associate itself with earlier claims about the solidaristic nature of the welfare state. Broad social services like universal healthcare have been claimed to boost or at least enhance solidarity.[13] Yet the relationship between population, statistics, and solidarity raises important questions with regard to social organization and how we understand community.

Of course, solidarity is a famously amorphous concept.[14] Here I will define solidarity as a disposition or virtue: "a firm and persevering determination to commit oneself to the common good."[15] It is a disposition similar to what Aristotle calls civic friendship, a well-wishing to the other that arises from a shared purpose and a shared work.[16] That is why it is so characteristically located in groups who engage in shared labor, such as unions or guilds.[17] The common good that is aimed at is not a statistical description of the population. It is not an aggregation of individual external goods like health or wealth, as one finds in the population vision. Instead, the common good includes shared purposes and a form of social relationship that arises from the joint pursuit of these internal goods. Solidarity is the concrete attachment that supports the participation of all in seeking this common end. This older ideal of solidarity contrasts with the solidarity oriented toward statistical measures found in preventive medicine. To see why this is important, this chapter will first discuss the problems of focusing on preventing the deaths of statistical lives over curing the diseases of identifiable others. It will then discuss how the statistical vision warps solidarity.

STATISTICAL LIVES AND IDENTIFIED LIVES

In public health and public policy discussions, the conflict that I describe as between statistical and concrete others is known as the debate between saving statistical lives and saving identified lives.[18] It is really a debate between prevention and cure. A commonly used example of the problem involves a mine rescue: Why should we spend millions rescuing thirty-three trapped mine workers when the same amount would save many more lives if spent on safety improvements that prevent mine accidents in the future? The question comes down to whether to prioritize the lives of the individual mine workers who are currently trapped over all the possible future people who, statistically, could be saved by a preventive intervention. Another thought experiment concerns a limited dose of medicine that will cure a disease if it is used in its entirety but, if given in small doses, will prophylactically prevent a disease. Should we prioritize saving the life of the currently sick person or preventing illness in the first place? Where do our commitments lie: to saving the currently suffering or to preventing the abstract possibility of future suffering?

Economists, public policy analysts, and other utilitarians have generally argued that there is no difference between statistical and identified lives. A life is a life in their equations. There is no reason for any preference between individuals. All that matters is maximizing the lives saved in the population. Any problems of future uncertainty (i.e., how do we know preventive measures will actually save lives?) can be factored into their equations.

Note how this position embodies the aspects of preventive medicine described in earlier chapters. It makes future possible harms equivalent to present disease. The possible dangers to future individuals exist in the real present. Those who embrace saving statistical lives are committed to denying the distinctions between present and future or actual versus possible.[19] Moreover, this framework indulges in abstraction from the person that one confronts. A person with a disease or trapped in a mine must be seen as part of a population of many such deaths, abstracting from the concrete suffering of their situation.

The most commonly recognized objections to equating statistical and identifiable lives draw on the impossibility or at least the dreadful effects of performing this effort of abstraction. Objectors point to the empathy elicited by immediate suffering,[20] or to a psychologically driven "rule of rescue" that impels us to respond to emergencies.[21] It would be harmful to medical care to have doctors who engaged their suffering patients in an abstract way and, instead of responding to their illness, judged them in terms of their cost with regard to population metrics.[22] Moreover, rejecting the priority of identifiable lives might undermine communal solidarity,[23] because solidarity is built upon practices of commitment toward concrete others.[24] Solidarity depends on the belief that others will support you in suffering, even at cost to themselves.[25] A focus on the statistical to the detriment of the actual can undermine solidarity, so overly focusing on prevention will not build solidarity.

Prevention and the Denial of Care

Emphasizing prevention over cure can also serve as an excuse to focus on economic goods to the exclusion of the real suffering of the marginalized. To see possible outcomes of the elevation of the statistical over the concrete, one need only consider the example of the debate over prevention versus treatment of HIV.[26] By the late 1990s, the advent of antiretroviral drugs such as AZT had made HIV into something more like a manageable chronic disease than the immediate death sentence that it had been early in the epidemic. Yet the epidemic raged unchecked through the Global South. Given the expense of antiretrovirals, global health agencies had chosen not to use them in low-income countries. Instead, they pursued a strategy of prevention: education, testing, condoms, and so forth. Many experts argued that prevention was much more cost-effective than treatment, saving more lives per dollar spent.[27] Global health agencies were also concerned about the capacity of local health systems to adequately distribute these medications and whether there was sufficient health literacy in the infected population to ensure compliance. Thus the identified lives of those dying from HIV were sacrificed to the statistical lives saved by prevention.

Paul Farmer, an infectious disease doctor working in Haiti, along with many others, rejected this choice. He thought it was a moral imperative to treat those who could be saved by available medication. Moreover, he found the economic analysis supporting prevention efforts to be naïve. If structural conditions like poverty are the root cause of HIV's spread in the Global South, then education will do no good in the face of ongoing poverty, violence against women, or the need to earn money from sex work. People's choices are too limited in conditions of extreme poverty. Further, sexual violence and the complex nature of patronage and sexual exchange would undermine condom distribution.[28] No one would seek testing if there were no treatment, since a positive result would lead only to anxiety and stigma. The realistic, hard-nosed approach embodied in cost-effectiveness is in fact founded in illusion—ultimately a cruel illusion.

To confront claims that antiretrovirals could not be effectively used in resource-poor settings, the organization Farmer cofounded, Partners in Health, initiated a demonstration project in Haiti. They showed that HIV could be effectively controlled in the Global South given the resources. This demonstration, along with Farmer's moral clarity, helped to push the international community toward HIV treatment in the early 2000s. Through initiatives like PEPFAR and the Global Fund, the world dramatically expanded antiretroviral treatment. Farmer showed the rationality and morality of treating identified over statistical lives.

Bare Life and Community

Even when medical practitioners engage actual patients, however, they can still do so under the form of a statistical vision. Abstraction is encouraged by the computerized decision support systems tied to reimbursement rates discussed in chapter 7. Through them, institutions encourage the doctor or nurse practitioner to view the patient only in terms of whether the appropriate medication is prescribed to reduce population health risk. Given the short length of most appointments, practitioners have little chance to grasp the social and personal world of the patient. They have time to see them only in terms of physiological risk factors. Thus patients can become statistical lives to the practitioner even when they sit directly in front of her. When viewed from the population perspective, the person is abstracted from all the social aspects of his life. He becomes merely vital statistics, like life span, denuded of community. He is understood only in terms of his animal, biological life, what some call bare life.[29]

This changed vision of the patient can have real effects. It can, as earlier chapters described, lead to overtreatment and to attempts at risk reduction that are completely inappropriate to the patient's goals and lived experience. It can also lead to great cruelty in the guise of care. Most obviously, this cruelty occurred in the case of those who were institutionalized during the pandemic. To curtail the spread of the virus, nursing homes and hospitals were almost completely quarantined. Visits from outside relatives and friends were curtailed, residents could not interact with each other, staff engagement was reduced, no one could leave. The dying were denied the comfort of loved ones and the spiritual solace of last rites. Residents' social worlds were eliminated, all in an effort to extend biological life, or to reduce the risk to bare life. Paradoxically, the elderly and dying were socially abandoned out of statistical solidarity. This situation and its aftermath exemplify the potential cruelty of statistical care.

—   Far from enhancing solidarity, the population perspective of preventive medicine can serve to undermine community. In its wake, others become objects of fear or ghostly statistical abstractions. Care for the immediately suffering is deferred to benefit future possible lives. This is not to say that addressing the suffering other does not have its dangers: it can lead to burnout; unwise and extreme efforts can be used, especially in end-of-life situations; and people can be reduced to simply the role of a suffering stranger.[30] Still, engaging concrete others in their suffering opens the possibility of encountering a real person and providing aid.[31]

Part III

Addressing the Problems

of Prevention

ELEVEN

Prevention and the Social Determinants of Health

If, as the first section of the book argued, the current regime of preventive health in which precision medicine is embedded causes significant medical side effects, and if its internal tendency is to ever intensify, grasping for more control and leading to ever more alienation, as the second section discussed, is prevention a retrievable goal? I would argue yes, but only with a changed approach to prevention. Prevention's general aim of reducing suffering from disease and death is good. My criticism addresses only a specific form of prevention, the medical management of population risk based in quantitative prediction of individual risk with no lower bounds. In this form, medicine seeks not merely those at high risk but tries to search out hidden risk of whatever level. It is the present medical paradigm that threatens to cause more problems than it solves. Dangers arise out of its specific form of broad screening and risk-reducing medication. Prevention is not worth the cost of bringing the experience of illness into the present. It is not worth medicalizing lives and social problems. It is not worth degrading social ties through abstraction and control. Small potential adjustments to future suffering are not worth making lives miserable in the present. Thankfully, we do not have to sacrifice the present for possible futures.

The last section of the book analyzes modes of prevention that do not entail medicalization. This chapter and the next will address structural factors that increase risk of disease in a population, things like the food or transportation systems. Instead of expanding the use of pharmaceuticals or nudging individual choices in response to quantitative risk analysis, our primary goal should be shifting social and cultural conditions to allow a healthier lifestyle. Interventions should address structures rather than individual risk. A structural strategy would seek to change the regularities inherent in both broad social conditions and the rhythms of daily life. Importantly, though, changing these social features is not the role of medicine. Social institutions and individual lifestyles must aim at other goods aside from reduced health risk, such as a general goal of justice or individual flourishing.

The last two chapters will address another strategy for prevention that aims only to address high-risk individuals with highly effective therapies, suggesting that very targeted prevention efforts may escape some of the problems discussed in chapter 2. Such a strategy can even positively use genetics and Big Data in identifying and treating ill and high-risk individuals. Further, by turning away from a need for intensive optimization, medicine can care for those whose risks cannot be controlled rather than rejecting them, which is the topic of the last chapter. This framework will allow for a nondestructive prevention.

Throughout these chapters, I hope to offer suggestions for what kinds of programs are open or resistant to the dangers of prevention based in the medical management of populations. I use these examples not because I know they are effective and think that people should implement them exactly as they currently exist. Their efficacy is a matter for empirical testing and description. They merely demonstrate the kinds of initiatives that embody the ethical perspective described here. These chapters aim to paint a picture of a different form of medicine that escapes the technocratic control and anxiety of its current instantiation.

Social Determinants of Health and the Limits of Medicine

Previous chapters have discussed a pharmaceutically driven model of shifting the population curve for risk factors: Treat the whole country with statins to bring down cardiovascular disease risk. Lower acceptable blood pressure guidelines and put broader and broader swaths of the country on antihypertensives. Diagnose more and more people with prediabetes and medicate accordingly. Expand the acceptable NNT of risk-reducing medications. The most astute advocates of preventive measures have long been suspicious of such strategies for many of the reasons discussed in this book: there is too little data on the potential long-term harms of these interventions, and the needed data are hard to gather.[1] Because knowledge of long-term harms is limited, any gains that one makes in life expectancy due to reduced cardiovascular disease or diabetes are in danger of being canceled out by small, unknown side effects of the medication. The dangers outweigh the benefits with any new compound or intervention that makes only small adjustments to risk.

Instead of adding new medicines, the epidemiologist Geoffrey Rose, one of the most prominent advocates of population strategies of preventive health, suggests removing things that increase risk that people have added to the human environment since the beginning of industrial modernity. Many risks come from new chemicals added to our environment or diet: cigarettes cause lung cancer; pollutants lead to asthma; high-fructose corn syrup allows for foods with the increased caloric density that lead to obesity; overconsumption of salt contributes to high blood pressure.[2] Over a long evolutionary and cultural history, human biology adjusted to many things in our environment. It is new things, what one might call "unnatural" things, that we have not adjusted to that lead to risks.[3] While due caution should be undertaken about the widespread use of any new material or intervention, efforts should also be taken to identify dangers that have already been introduced to the environment. This is where good population-level epidemiological work is so essential; it is difficult but crucial to determine the unintended consequences for human health of new additions to the environment. Thus I am not against statistical or public health research. It is extremely important. The problem is that public health research is drastically underdeveloped at this point, in part because of pressures from interests and ideological motivations. For example, the tobacco industry fought long and hard to obscure research on the harms of cigarettes.[4]

More importantly, we must change basic structural features of society. Epidemiologists have convincingly shown that the biggest effects on health and longevity come from social conditions, such as income inequality, food supply, or inadequate housing.[5] People in poverty generally have reduced life expectancy. Both inadequate food supply and, more likely today, a surfeit of unhealthy food lead to health problems. Society can shift the incidence of negative risk factors, but only by changing the broader culture, so public health and population health practitioners correctly identify the need to address underlying features of social institutions. The problem is that medical authorities have little expertise in shaping the fundamental features of society.

For example, job satisfaction is a factor that has one of the strongest impacts on longevity and health. Factors like low job control, job insecurity, and an imbalance between efforts and rewards lead to increased rates of coronary heart disease, diabetes, and mortality.[6] This is extremely important data and shows that we must improve our culture of work.[7] Yet what possible role could medicine or public health play in improving job satisfaction? Would doctors distribute surveys to continually monitor job satisfaction, or would they encourage programs or workshops on improving job satisfaction? From all of my experiences of HR-driven programs, such bureaucratic impositions would only lower job satisfaction. There is little that is more painful than sitting through expert-led attempts at team building. The satisfaction of work must be drawn from sources internal to its practice rather than merely manipulated by outside experts to reach external social ends. People must discover how to enhance the internal goods of work and vocation, something that the techniques of public health cannot do.

The danger is that the social determinants of health, which are in fact broad social and political problems, will become redefined as health problems. Admittedly, many policymakers may see turning social issues into health problems as the only way to address them. As discussed in chapter 6, in an individualist, utilitarian society like our own, too few citizens are concerned with broader issues of justice, especially if these may cause inconvenience to themselves. Everyone cares about health, though, especially if an intervention might serve to reduce the cost of healthcare, thus reducing their own insurance premiums and taxes. However, redefining social goals like the culture of work in terms of health inevitably brings social problems under the purview of medicine, which both alters *how* a problem is addressed and ultimately shifts the *ends* that are sought through interventions.

The goods tied to these social structures go far beyond medicine, so there is a danger that a medicalized understanding of social problems will reshape the ends sought in attempts to address them. To illustrate this concern, take the example of loneliness as described by the sociologist Joseph Davis.[8] Many commentators have noted an expanding problem of loneliness in contemporary society. The United Kingdom even went so far as to appoint a minister to take the lead on the loneliness problem. This loneliness epidemic has many causes: an aging society, family breakdown, individualism, and an increasing amount of time spent with technology, all made worse by the social isolation of the pandemic. People intuitively recognize that loneliness is a problem, but what is interesting is the way experts have justified government attention: the health effects of loneliness. For example, loneliness leads to stress, which leads to inflammation and cardiovascular risk; or it is a risk for mental health issues like depression. The problem of loneliness has thus been medicalized, and researchers are already using AI to detect it.[9] This medical focus then shapes potential solutions. For example, one set of researchers is working on a drug that can alleviate feelings of loneliness. Other solutions focus on forms of self-help or cognitive therapy that lead people to reinterpret their situation in order to better deal with the lack of intimate human relationships. Thus an individual can continue in social isolation without experiencing the health risks of heart attacks and depression. Yet such a solution completely misunderstands the problem. Social isolation is a problem *in itself* because humans are social, relational creatures. It is not just the health effects but the condition itself that is the problem. Even if it had no health effects, social isolation would be bad because it is a failure to enact a basic human good.

The problem is that the language of public health can misidentify problems, leading to mistargeted solutions. Using the language of health can lead us to treat symptoms rather than underlying moral problems. Loneliness is treated through pharmaceuticals rather than rebuilt communities. Substance abuse becomes the target of harm reduction through the broad availability of Narcan and clean needles, leaving people in the hell of addiction even while reducing mortality and morbidity rates. Heart disease arising from inequality is dealt with through risk-reducing medication rather than social change. It is much easier to turn to technocratic solutions once social problems are defined as health problems and health problems are managed through risk-reducing pharmaceuticals.

Medicalizing a problem also shifts who is thought of as capable of arranging a solution. Medicine requires an education in science followed by a long apprenticeship in practice. When a problem becomes medicalized, the barrier of expertise necessary for engagement with it becomes similar to that found in medicine. It becomes an expert concern, so entering the conversation requires a background in research, policy, or economics as well as long experience with an issue. Because of this demand for expertise, medicalization moves problems out of the public sphere.[10] The public problem is no longer something that lay people seem competent to address. Thus the problem moves out of the sphere of politics and the public square, and into the far more restricted circles of bureaucratic policy, or technocracy. It is removed from the hands of the local and placed into the hands of small circles at higher levels of government and healthcare corporations.

It would be foolish to be reflexively antiexpertise, since such a restriction to expertise makes sense in many fields that require engaging a specific body of technical data. It is more questionable in relation to the social determinants of health, though. By their very nature, these are problems that affect the whole of society. They are issues of wealth distribution, food policy, or transportation. These are fundamentally political problems dealing with which ends society should prioritize. We frequently think of politics today in terms of division and conflict over political power, but I am using the term here in the older Aristotelian and civic republican sense of matters of broad shared concern that should be solved by engaging the citizenry as a whole in common discussion. These problems need to be addressed through such political engagement, as difficult as this may seem in our current political climate.

If health policymakers bypass politics, then their interventions will face two possible reasons for failure. First, they will lack the requisite means to truly address the problem. Fundamental issues of social organization can be addressed only through solutions that have a broad social legitimacy. This legitimacy can be brought about only through the political process. It makes no difference if we develop effective Covid vaccines if large numbers of people refuse to get the shot. Well-developed plans of social distancing are useless if people flout the rules. Furthermore, one might not be able to muster sufficient material means to address a large social problem without the backing of widespread support. One sees this issue in contemporary responses to the social determinants of health like housing. Instead of addressing the political economic problem of the high cost of housing in urban areas, a problem that surely will require a multi-faceted response, medicalized responses such as those frequently on offer by population health programs target only a few high-risk patients. They might provide housing vouchers or place some homeless people in hotel rooms, or perhaps a health system might help build a set of apartments for some of its patients. These are responses that, while good for some individuals, will not truly address the problem of housing.

To take a different example, medicalization shifts the political question of how our food system should be organized to a technical question of targeted intervention. Numerous authors have traced the current problems of obesity to government policy: for example, subsidies for corn that lead to an artificially low price for high-fructose corn syrup.[11] Our agricultural policy has further enabled the centralization of farming into a few hands, a concentration of land that allows for industrial monocropping. Addressing such structural features of our food system requires extensive political engagement of the kind that a purely medical approach does not allow. Instead, medicalization leads to far more limited interventions: a few urban gardens, maybe a low-priced cooperative grocery store, more likely some food vouchers. Medicalization ironically shifts the focus away from the need for structural reform that was at the heart of the social determinants of health approach into a much narrower range of technical solutions.

By moving these issues into the medical, and thus expert, realm, generally also a realm coordinated according to data analytics, policymakers make it impossible for local agencies and voluntary groups to participate. Expert analysis frequently works at an abstract, quantitative, generalized level. Such analyses, while valuable and revealing in their own right, can obscure specific problems of context and individual variation. Social scientists have repeatedly cautioned us about the way that the bureaucratic gaze can oversimplify problems,[12] especially since these problems are going to be affected by the specificity of a context. To take a simple example, the food crisis in Appalachia will take a different form than in urban Chicago, and the solutions will also differ. The housing crisis in the urban tech hub of San Francisco will take a different shape than that in the small college town of Charlottesville. Engaging local organizations enables local knowledge to be brought to bear on a problem.

Someone might object that usually population health programs do use nongovernmental and community organizations (NGOs) in order to allow participation and engage local knowledges. Many population health advocates are insistent on the need for health systems to partner with other kinds of local groups.[13] Partnerships could solve these problems, but in practice NGOs are less free from expert control than they might seem. To function and act, they require grants from government or business. As much research on NGOs has shown, these organizations are forced to reshape their priorities and programs in order to align them with funding calls.[14] An NGO will not get the grant if its programs do not match the form prescribed by a request for proposals. These requests are themselves written to meet the best practices set forth by expert knowledge. Thus the aim of engaging local knowledge and local participation is frequently defeated because local actors are subtly pressured to conform to the priorities of those with power and money, even when those in power have good intentions.

Further, insurance companies and health systems might not be the best organizations to address problems like housing because their interests are obviously, and appropriately, narrower. They aim to help their specific patients and reduce their own costs. Moreover, they should not have to address these problems in their totality. Just because an issue is medically relevant does not mean that it is the responsibility of the medical system. After all, we do not look to hospitals to provide a city with clean water and sanitation, even though these play a far greater role in promoting health and extending life span than anything medicine does.

Does this mean the medical system has no role to play? Of course not. The social determinants of health are indeed medically relevant, so healthcare systems should engage with other stakeholders to address root causes. This should be done broadly through the political system, not just narrowly through health experts, with health systems making their voices heard in larger policy discussions. A health system should engage local organizations, but not in ways that overshadow their ability for independent action. Action should focus on broad social goods rather than narrower metrics. These are harder things to do than might first appear. It would be second nature for public health experts to address health metrics through forms of bureaucratic best practices. These would be neither the most just nor the most effective way to proceed, though. Healthcare systems must engage other stakeholders. Organizations and actors that are not specifically focused on health are much less likely to examine the problem from the point of view of health alone, thus preventing the problems of medicalization.

—   All the data on the social determinants of health indicate the desperate need for changes in culture and social structure. Yet once we turn our gaze in this direction, medicine and public health play little role. These are problems for politics and social ethics that can be worked out only in the public sphere. Moreover, such changes must be directed toward justice and the internal goods of the various practices at issue. Medicine can play merely a supporting role.[15]

It is important to emphasize that political responses to the social determinants of health do not evince the two major problems of precision and preventive medicine. They do not bring one's own future illness into present awareness. Nor do they attempt to manipulate the individual as a part of a population. Instead, they attempt to change structural conditions. They try to develop an alternative vision of our shared social life through politics rather than expertise. Most importantly, they should focus on the internal goods of human practices rather than external goods of efficiency and risk.

TWELVE

Regimen

Though shifts in structural features of society could contribute to the improvement of health, much will still ultimately depend on individual action. Although the wealthier are on average healthier, even a well-to-do person can overeat, drink too much, or fail to exercise. Looking at such health activities as exercise or proper diet in terms of discrete occasions of success or failure is not sufficient, though. Health depends on healthy habits, or rather a healthy lifestyle.[1] Ancient writing on health focused primarily on creating a set of habits or a schedule for one's day that encompassed eating, bathing, exercise, and work. These various habits were brought together under the name of regimen, a rule of life. In this way, shifting individual habits also depends on changing structures, albeit the structures of one's own life.

In older forms of medicine, the person promotes her own health primarily by adopting the proper regimen.[2] Hippocratic and Galenic medicine had few tools to treat diseases. Some of the most popular involved specialized diets based on their theories of bodily humors and individual disposition.[3] Illness came from an overabundance or lack of one of the four humors, and thus it could be resolved by adjusting diet, purging excess humors, or taking one of the medications that affected the humors. Since disease came about from humoral dysregulation, preventive efforts aimed at ensuring a continuous balance of the humors. A regimen was a certain form of life, regular practices of eating, sleeping, exercising, dress, even sex, that contributed to health. This form of life was adapted to the individual constitution, age, and occupation of the patient as well as to the climate of his locality and the season of the year. The patient was to eat certain things in winter, change sleeping patterns in response to illness, exercise differently at different stages of life, and so on. Diet, exercise, and a regularity attuned to the patient's bodily dispositions and the seasons became tools for ensuring health. It was a total style of life.

In this attention to diet and exercise, there is a continuity and perhaps a deeper truth to the wellness framework. Many wellness programs encourage exercise and healthy eating. Public policy nudges likewise attempt to decrease consumption of sugars and fatty foods in favor of fruits and vegetables. They, along with many doctors, attempt to decrease health risk by transforming people's lives. This way of addressing health risk converges with perennial themes of medicine and philosophy: protecting health by transforming habits.

Yet there are two sets of limitations to this approach as it exists today. The first set is pragmatic: we lack the proper knowledge and social structures to truly allow people to take charge of their regimen. The second is philosophical. Medical attention to regimen can make it too exclusively focused on health. Traditionally, most people have attended to regimen to help them achieve a broader set of goals, with health serving as a subordinate aim that assists in realizing other ends in their life. Indeed, some regimens allow for damage to health if that is necessary. Medical regimen, though, is likely to overemphasize health, possibly leading to a morbid obsession or a paralyzing fear of death. People can spend all their time tinkering with aspects of diet or exercise. This chapter explores how to avoid these different sorts of problems.

Pragmatic Concerns with Contemporary Regimens

The most basic problem of contemporary, or even ancient, medical regimens is that they tend to treat food in the same way that we treat risk-reducing pharmaceuticals.[4] The phenomenon of nutraceuticals and superfoods is perhaps the clearest example of this. Oddly enough, many people replace regulated pharmaceuticals for unregulated chemical supplements as a way to be more natural, though taking a processed pill, especially one whose ingredients may not be what the consumer expects, is not especially natural. Even the nutritional information box on most foods leads in this direction. Food becomes chemistry, a mix of partially hydrogenated fats, differently sourced sugars, protein, vitamins, and preservatives. The aim becomes balancing different intakes in the most healthful way. Food is engaged as the material that keeps the body as machine running. In this model of diet, anything can be eaten at any time as long as the chemical components are balanced in a way that reduces risk.

This reductionist culinary framework can lead to a morbid obsession with health and diet. The person continually counts calories and quantifies nutrients. Anxiety over future disease can influence every meal. Or after a failure to properly address food as risk, regret and guilt assails the person. Risk becomes a task to address episodically at each mealtime, which prevents the formation of a true regimen, a habitual form of life, that the person can engage without ongoing choice. Diet can become merely a version of the risk paradigm that is not mediated through pharmaceuticals.

Moreover, we lack the knowledge to execute risk reduction through food. Whatever my concerns about pharmaceutical research, our knowledge of nutrition is at a far more rudimentary level. It is nearly impossible research to conduct. One would have to ensure that thousands of people maintained a prescribed diet for years if not decades. It is simply unimaginable to maintain that kind of discipline among a large, voluntary study population. Observational studies are filled with errors and confounding factors. If researchers try to observe different groups with different diets (e.g., Okinawans vs. Kansans), they are confronted by the problem of dealing with the confounding effects of all the other aspects of life that differ between these populations. If they try to track diet through self-reports, they are left with data that is widely recognized as inaccurate; people too often forget or misrepresent what they eat. Despite its importance, we lack much of the basic knowledge necessary for a precision diet.

Finally, adopting a proper regimen is possible only if the structures of society allow for it. Ancient regimens brought other actors besides medicine into the promotion of health. Foremost among these has been the state, which shapes the structural constraints of the individual regimen. It, along with civil society, helps to shape the human ecology that enables a good form of life. Classical philosophy recognized the importance of civic institutions for preserving a good regimen. For example, many of Plato's

Laws concern setting up social ground rules (land size, military service) that promoted health and virtue.[5] Perhaps the most important aspect is ensuring that policies do not undermine healthy regimens. For a recent example, heavy investment in the highway system rather than mass transit in the 1950s promoted the growth of suburbs, which in turn promoted a regimen that did not include physical activity as a daily part of life, such as walking to work. Instead, people were forced into driving and thus needed to set aside special periods for intensive exercise. Similarly, subsidies for corn decrease the price of high-fructose corn syrup and corn feed, decreasing the price of sweets and meat.[6] No similar support is given for fruits and vegetables. Such considerations need to be a greater part of public deliberation. As chapter 11 argued, changes in social structure are necessary for many people to be able to take true responsibility for their health.

A factor that is even more difficult to address comes from the cultural meaning of food. Different social classes' distinct diets are part of their self-understanding. Pierre Bourdieu chronicled the reasons behind the particular diets of workers and bourgeoisie in 1960s France.[7] While some of the differences in eating patterns arose simply from the prices of food, many of them resulted from different meanings that food held for different classes. The working-class meal was "characterized by plenty . . . and above all by freedom,"[8] with abundant, fatty dishes, like stews, that nourished. It emphasized the material reality of eating.[9] In contrast, a light diet, like fish, reflected a bourgeois obsession with self-control and refinement.[10] Changing a diet requires changing the cultural meanings that surround food. For the individual, this might even mean taking on a new identity. Optimal health is rarely a sufficient reason for such dramatic changes.

Philosophical Concerns with Medical Regimens

There is a deeper problem with regimen as risk reduction, though. It is that people might shape their whole life around resisting death. Take, for example, the inventor, futurist, and transhumanist Ray Kurzweil. Every day, he consumes 180 to 210 supplements. He spends one day a week receiving intravenous (potentially) longevity-enhancing treatments.[11] His diet, his whole life, is aimed at staving off death in the hope that he might survive until the day when technology allows people to live forever.[12] On the one hand, this concern over resisting death undermines courage. Ancient philosophers were clear that the only way to live a life of freedom and truth was to come to terms with death.[13] That was the reason that the *memento mori* was such a central practice in ancient, medieval, and early modern spirituality. Without accepting the reality of death, a person will be constantly haunted by anxiety over his ultimate demise. Moreover, he will fail to make the courageous, risky choices necessary to live in the truth because of his fear of death.[14] A routine of life focused solely on avoiding death cannot but undermine the courage necessary for a good life.

Plato was concerned about rich citizens spending all their lives grasping after the correct medical regimen for a slightly different reason.[15] He thought health a too narrow goal for which to live and one that distracts the person from the common good. In part, this rejection of intensive regimen is due to Plato's problematic rejection of people with disabilities and chronic diseases. Yet that such concerns are not just due to early eugenic sensibilities is seen in Galen's criticism of athletic training regimens, which seemed to disqualify wrestlers and others from ordinary military activity for the *polis*.[16] Even though the athlete lives at peak performance, the limited focus of his training makes him useless to the common good. The deeper problem that these authors identify is that a regimen ordered only to bodily goods like health can distract a person from richer ends. Philosophers in antiquity, while recognizing the value of medicine and health, criticized the totalizing tendencies of ancient medicine, its capacity, even in antiquity, to make health the primary end of all activity.[17]

Even among those engaged in the Quantified Self (QS) movement, we see this desire for a richer end than mere survival. QSers are people committed to some kind of digital self-tracking, as described in chapter 1. Much of this tracking aims at health information. Yet not all of it. Some QS enthusiasts track their mood, their interactions with others, or various aspects of their daily routines.[18] Many of them admit that they do not seek mere health but instead track their emotions and how they respond to specific situations. Their true aim is self-knowledge. They may be engaging this quest in a deeply mistaken way, because true self-knowledge does not come through quantitative readouts. But, for many of them, their activity aims at a goal that is deeper than mere survival or risk reduction.

Ancient philosophers also aimed at a goal beyond mere health. The goal of a regimen was to allow for the philosophical life.[19] Such a life is impossible if one is consumed by the desires encouraged by intemperance, so health was always a subsidiary good of practices that aimed just as much at perfecting the soul.[20] Simple eating improves health, but more importantly, it forms temperance. Drinking moderately supports health, but more importantly it avoids drunkenness while promoting conviviality. Contemplation is difficult if one is ill. Therefore, they aimed at a temperate, healthy regimen to enable their search for truth. They lived according to nature both physically and mentally, and they tried to control desires to allow for a life according to reason.

One of the first treatises on Christian ethics that we have, Clement of Alexandria's *Paidagogos*, concerns the shape of the Christian form of life.[21] In it, Clement justifies a certain kind of Christian regimen, one primarily aimed at an upper-class Christian audience to be sure, but with elements more broadly applicable. "As there is one sort of training for philosophers, another for orators and another for wrestlers, so, too, there is an excellent disposition imparted by the education of Christ.... As for deeds, walking and reclining at table, eating and sleeping, marriage relations and the manner of life, the whole of a man's education all become illustrious as holy deeds under the influence of the Educator."[22] Christians should eat plain food, because "Antiphanes, the Delian physician, has said that rich variety in food is one of the causes of disease," but also because culinary extravagance breeds gluttony and destroys charity.[23] Sleep aids digestion and relaxes the body, but Christians should limit sleep, waking to pray and keeping vigils for the Lord.[24] Bathing is good for health and cleanliness, but too much induces lassitude and becomes a source of unworthy pleasure.[25] Thus health is always one reason for choosing a course of life, but never the sole or even the most important one.

Later, Neoplatonic philosophers went further in allowing for the sacrifice of health to seek higher goods of contemplation.[26] These same goals, along with penitence, also animated Christian ascetics. For Thomas Aquinas, drawing on these Neoplatonic sources, naturally acquired temperance and temperance infused through grace have different measures with regard to eating: "The mean fixed by human reason, is that food should not harm the health of the body, nor hinder the use of reason: whereas, according to the Divine rule, it behooves man to 'chastise his body, and bring it into subjection' (1 Cor 9:27), by abstinence in food, drink, and the like."[27] Similarly, perfecting or purgative temperance, far from maximizing health, "so far as nature allows, neglects the needs of the body."[28] Higher goods came before health.

That health was a subordinate good is clear from the discussion of the obligation to care for health discussed in chapter 8. A person could continue in the discipline of a religious order, even if it was clear that such a discipline would shorten his life. He had joined a certain state, a form of life that is not in itself unhealthy, but just became so for his particular constitution. The ultimate goal sought by this form of life is so valuable, though, that a risk to health is appropriate.[29]

Of course, there are dangers to such asceticism. Intense quests for a more spiritual form of life run the danger of indulging a Gnostic hatred for the body that deliberately would destroy it. Many scholars fear asceticism because they tie it to bodily self-hatred or a desire for control like that seen in eating disorders.[30] The Desert Fathers, though, as described by John Cassian, were less concerned with Gnosticism than with pride. Ascetic lifestyles threatened to become a competition to demonstrate how much one could do without. Asceticism can overinvolve the practitioners in their lifestyles and achievements, causing them to lose sight of the practices' ultimate spiritual goal. Similarly, people today can become overly fixated on lifestyle and habit, on sharing their exercise regimens and healthy diets on social media. Regimen can become overly elaborated, almost dandyish.[31]

Christian and Neoplatonic philosophers, however, rejected both Gnosticism and pride. That is why the diets of Christian ascetics were brought under careful community control: to prevent self-destructive behaviors that could mark a prideful attempt to exalt oneself above others. Early monastic writing takes great care in determining which food to eat when.[32] A somewhat grueling diet aided in the monks' attempts to discipline their bodies to overcome temptations of lust and gluttony. A too restrictive diet, however, could damage health and, more troublingly, indicate pride.[33] A strict regimen avoided these contrasting dangers, leading, hopefully, to the virtue of temperance. Diet was essential to monks' achievement of their final end. That their regimen was not directed toward the destruction of the body is shown by their impressive developments in organized healthcare institutions that will be discussed in chapter 14. If monastics became ill, they were treated with richer diets; their regimen was adjusted accordingly.[34] Christian ascetics wanted to care for the body, which would rise with them on the last day, even if it was not their highest goal.

Even for the laity, fasting was brought under communal discipline. The community as a whole fasted on particular days, with Pope Leo arguing that the collective fast was more efficacious than individual efforts.[35] Fasting became part of a communal activity that aimed at a collective way of life. This social aspect of fasting reduced the dangers of pride and Gnosticism. It also generated communal solidarity. For these reasons, the loss of communal norms of abstinence and fasting impoverishes contemporary church efforts at a nondestructive asceticism.

—   For most paths of intentional life in the ancient Mediterranean, health would be one goal of a regimen that would exist primarily to enable the achievement of other goods. Established ascetic practices do not seem to noticeably impede life span.[36] Even so, a regimen would aim at health as a subordinate good. It would not be a highly targeted, reductionist focus on risk. Instead, a regimen would include a reshaped framework of habits in which diet and exercise would be a part. These individual habits, however, would be subsumed into a broader communal framework, with even individual Stoics sharing details of their regimen with friends. A regimen is social rather than individualized, allowing for the elaboration of shared cultural meanings around diet, exercise, and lifestyle that provides goods beyond mere temporal survival. It is at this kind of regimen that we must aim for a reshaped structure of individual life.

THIRTEEN

Genomics in the Identification and Treatment of Disease

Despite my criticisms of particular applications, the precision medicine technologies of genomics, AI, and Big Data have many positive uses in the clinic beyond prevention. Genetic therapies for felt disease are now entering the clinic. Over the last decade, the FDA has approved several therapies for single-gene disorders, such as hemophilia and spinal muscular atrophy. New genetic technologies like CRISPR are promising further treatments for diseases like sickle cell anemia. Here we see the realization of the dreams of pre–Human Genome Project genetics coming to fruition in the repair of discrete genetic disorders. The question is whether postgenomic technologies will also see this kind of success.

There is nothing about these technologies that inevitably ties them to the project of indefinitely reducing risk and the induction of suspicion about the body that is the target of my critique. In fact, they have great roles to play in the clinic in treating felt disease and in restoring health defined as the absence of disease. They even can play a role in limiting the scope of clinical analysis of risk by identifying especially high-risk patients. This chapter will delineate these two areas in which the technologies of precision medicine avoid some of the problems discussed in previous chapters.

Ending the Diagnostic Odyssey

Many common genetic conditions are easily diagnosed by medical practitioners, such as Down syndrome. In such cases, practitioners will know which tests will give a clear diagnosis. For other children, the diagnostic process does not proceed so smoothly. Many genetic conditions are highly variable, not always appearing in the same way. Their severity is mitigated by environmental conditions or other genes, which is called incomplete penetrance. In some patients, the problem is that the condition is rare, appearing only once in a hundred thousand or million births. Some conditions may have only a few cases in the world. General practitioners will not recognize them; perhaps only a few specialists would. In such unclear situations, it may even be doubtful as to whether the disease is genetic at all: perhaps the child was deprived of oxygen during birth, perhaps there was an infection, perhaps she was placed face down in the crib. Parents can face nightmares of potential responsibility with its resulting feelings of guilt.

When the causes of a condition are unclear, parents are forced to embark on what many call a diagnostic odyssey: referred to specialist after specialist; endlessly searching the internet for clues; becoming experts in obscure medical literature; observing the child for any additional symptom that would be the key to unlocking the mystery; asking friends for recommendations; enduring test after test.[1] Only upon having a diagnosis is there a possibility that their child will receive adequate treatment. The process is long, slow, stressful, and frustrating.

In such situations, genomics can bring relief. By sequencing and analyzing the child's genome, researchers can bring to light mutations that may cause the condition. For example, as part of the British 100,000 Genomes Project, researchers performed whole-genome sequencing on 4,660 patients with an undiagnosed disease that was suspected to have a genetic component.[2] They obtained diagnoses in 25 percent of the cases. These diagnoses may have been a major relief, since the median length of the diagnostic odyssey for these patients was seventy-five months, including a median sixty-eight hospital visits.[3] Finally, after such a long time, a subset of patients and their families knew their conditions. In the best-case scenario, there are treatments for the condition that can at least ameliorate the symptoms the child faces. In the project described above, 25 percent of the diagnoses were immediately clinically actionable. Even if there are no treatments, at least the parents' diagnostic odyssey, and resulting uncertainty, are brought to an end, which is a relief to many.

Precision medicine is not a panacea for these patients. After all, it succeeded in only a quarter of the cases. In other patients, the condition may not be genetic, in which case the diagnostic odyssey continues. Even worse, the results of the genomic analysis may not be clear. Sometimes no known mutation appears, just DNA sequences that differ from the standard genetic sequence. Perhaps there is a base pair that is different from what is common in the population, but this variant is not clearly related to making a protein defective or inoperative. Such differences are called variants of unknown significance (VUSs). It is uncertain whether the VUS is actually the cause of any conditions. Thus parents may be left with only the suspicion of a cause but no assurance, and certainly no treatment.

Even if a known mutation is identified, it may not result in better health for the child. Perhaps there is no treatment. Worse, perhaps the treatments are too expensive for the parents to afford, with, for example, a treatment for a retinal disease costing $425,000 per eye, a treatment for spinal muscular atrophy costing $2.1 million, a treatment for beta-thalassemia costing $2.8 million per patient, and a $3.5 million hemophilia treatment.[4] These therapies are so expensive that some have been withdrawn from European countries because of cost.[5] Even the pharmaceuticals for some conditions can be very expensive. Knowledge of a genetic cause may not lead to treatment for a patient and may even lead to parents realizing that their child is excluded from treatment because of a lack of resources.

Even when there is no treatment for a disease, however, such genomic analysis can still bring benefits of both tangible and intangible kinds. When I was in graduate school, a geneticist visited our lab and shared with us why he found working on rare genetic conditions so rewarding, even if this work was still far from finding cures: it was the calls from parents grateful that he was even working on these diseases. The parents were thankful for the knowledge that put an end to their diagnostic odyssey. More importantly, they were heartened to know that someone was working on their child's problem; they were not alone, someone else cared enough to devote their research career to their child's condition. The parents became aware of broader networks of solidarity in their struggles.

It opens other avenues for solidarity as well. With the internet, parents can connect to others whose children experience the same disorder.[6] Such connections can lead to more tangible benefits for their child. Parents learn what ameliorative therapies worked for others in similar situations and gain support during hard times. They do not have to follow the medical literature on their own but can be updated by others. Such groups can even band together to support research or advocacy efforts.[7] There is thus much to cheer in this form of precision medicine, even if it will not bring about miracle cures. However, it is important to temper our expectations for what this research can accomplish.

Sequencing Tumors and Cancer Care

Another field that demonstrates the value of precision medicine technologies is cancer, because it is in part a genetic disease. The most prominent theories of cancer depict it as occurring after mutations occur in multiple genes regulating the division and identity of cells. Instead of staying put and performing their normal function, cancer cells start dividing, change their shape, and begin to move. The cells' regulatory machinery, losing genes or being overwhelmed by mutant genes encouraging multiplication, ceases to function. The cells stop taking orders and begin to threaten the rest of the body.

Sometimes these genetic mutations are congenital. Most cancers, though, are not due to any singular genetic cause. Even in the case of breast cancer, genetic predisposing factors like BRCA1 and BRCA2 mutations account for only 5 to 10 percent of cases.[8] That means a DTC genomic test would falsely put the majority of potential breast cancer cases at ease. Mutations are still implicated in these other cases, just not hereditary mutations. All through our lives, our cells are suffering mutations from a variety of sources: UV radiation from sun exposure (skin cancer); environmental toxins (such as smoking and lung cancer); mistakes in the regular copying of our genome as cells divide throughout our lives. Even in people with congenital mutations, such as people with BRCA1 mutations, tumors are due to mutations in other genes that arise over the course of one's life. Not every cell in the breast becomes cancerous, only ones in which additional mutations occur. Not even everyone with a BRCA1 mutation gets breast cancer. Much depends on these chance mutations.

Because these diseases are genetic, medicine can use genetics to address them. Practitioners can zero in on the proteins that are causing the uncontrolled division and survival of cells in particular tumors. Over the past few decades, it has become apparent that the tissue classifications that have been used to define cancer types (breast, pancreatic, lung, skin, etc.) are far too broad. Armed with increasing genetic knowledge, oncologists are realizing that perhaps each tumor is different, caused by a distinct set of mutations with a unique history. Genomics might allow caregivers insight into individual tumors so that they can design tailored treatments.

The first genetically tailored treatments emerged in the 1980s, when researchers attempted to develop drugs against specific genes that cause cancer. One of the most famous examples is Herceptin.[9] Researchers discovered that HER2, a cell surface protein that receives signals that stimulate growth, is present in many breast cancer tumors. They developed a monoclonal antibody, Herceptin, that inhibits HER2 and found that its use could extend the life of women whose tumors showed increased presence of HER2. Now most women who are diagnosed with breast cancer are tested for the presence of HER2 (along with estrogen and progesterone receptors, two other proteins that can lead to cell growth and division). If the tests are positive, the patients will be prescribed a course of Herceptin along with their other treatment.

Herceptin is a remarkable success story, but there are only a few other examples of the development of a targeted drug with such broad applicability, such as Gleevec. The initial high expectations for this tailored research strategy have not come to fruition as a universal approach to curing disease. Either commonly mutated genes have been resistant to research efforts or there is too little commonality among genes expressed in different tumors. Because of these problems, as well as the decreasing cost of sequencing, a new paradigm has emerged in oncology over the past decade. If each tumor is unique, and the cells in the tumor are different, then perhaps doctors should sequence the tumors themselves. At some cancer institutes, researchers have begun sequencing the genomes of tumor cells. Through this process, they seek the specific mutations that are active in a particular tumor. From this information, they hope to find mutated genes for which pharmaceutical treatments already exist.[10] If an obvious drug is not found, the goal is to develop a large enough database so that they will be able to see what treatment regimens were effective in similar tumors. Here we see an ideal deployment of the principles of precision medicine: using genomics to access the particular causes of an individual's disease in order to design a targeted treatment regimen.

There are problems, though. Such approaches are expensive. Though advances in sequencing technology and data analytics may bring down costs in the future, these steps are still costly for the individual patient, although perhaps not in relation to the broader cost of cancer treatment.[11] There will always be the need for expert analysis, which itself costs money, and its expense tends to rise rather than shrink over time. The development of these targeted drugs is expensive and time-consuming, and these costs are passed on to the patients. Since markets in these areas tend not to be large, the cost of each individual treatment course is high.

Even ignoring costs, there are questions of efficacy.[12] Sequencing a tumor will not always identify a good treatment regimen; in fact it seems that it somewhat rarely does. A recent review of clinical trials for drugs that targeted multiple tumor types that shared the same genetic marker found on average only a 23 percent response rate.[13] This response rate varied widely according to tumor and genetic marker. Targeted drugs do not work against every tumor. Even when they do work, their benefits in terms of added life may be counted in weeks or months rather than years. At the same time, all of these treatments have side effects that can lead to lower quality of life during those additional months of life. Because of such side effects, many studies have shown that patients tend to live longer when placed in hospice than when they get aggressive cancer treatment. Again, precision oncology is no panacea, but it may lead to benefits in individual cases.

Though these sequencing technologies show some promise, it is not clear how well they work. Surely some of their appeal is just the hype surrounding the novel. They will all need rigorous testing. And here is also where statistical testing in terms of populations plays a role. Well-designed clinical trials are crucial for discovering whether treatments actually work. Because of the vast number of combinations of genetic markers, diagnostic tests, tumor types, and therapeutics, it will require a significant, coordinated research effort to clarify which options are effective.[14] Too often, though, clinical trials are shoddily done in order to speed approval of the drug or intervention. Data are massaged; healthier than usual test subjects are used; inappropriate controls are run; small effect sizes are trumpeted as significant.[15] Better trial design, oversight, and analysis can address these problems. Even when trials are well done, there is no coordinated effort that will ensure effectiveness. Solving these problems will require much-needed changes at the FDA and other regulatory bodies. Thus I am far from being against statistical analysis in medical research, despite the impression one might have gotten in this book. What is needed is more and better statistical analysis of our interventions.

Addressing the High Risk

Another area in which these technologies can be useful regards those at especially high risk. There are indeed many risks that do need to be addressed in the clinic. As I noted in the first chapter, some kinds of risk that arise outside the gaze of medicine can impinge upon one's feeling of dwelling in the body. If a woman's mother, sister, great-aunt, and cousin all die of breast cancer, the risk of breast cancer will be felt as a semiactualized possibility in her life. She will feel ill at ease knowing that the possibility exists. If a man's father, grandfather, and uncle all died of heart attacks in their fifties, he will view his own heart with suspicion, waiting for the day it will betray him. Neither of these examples of suspicion of the body arises from the pressures of medicine. These are the kinds of fears that arise out of daily life and family history.

Medicine should address these kinds of high-risk patients, and precision medicine has tools to help them. There are clear cases where an intensive focus on risk reduction makes sense, such as statins for people with hypercholesterolemia or increased breast cancer screening for women with a familial history of cancer and the BRCA1 mutation. By addressing high-risk individuals who are in the top, say, 10 percent of those at risk, medicine gets a much lower NNT. The epidemiologist Geoffrey Rose prefers the strategy of changing population structures because it would prevent a far larger number of deaths. He is probably right in his preference. Yet if we want to determine the role of precision medicine in the clinic, it is this: finding situations in which medical treatment leads to major benefits in addressing high-risk individuals.[16]

Yet even though risk management technologies can do much good, they are exposed to the dangerous tendency to indefinitely expand their reach discussed in chapter 6. Their implementation threatens to undermine independent clinical judgment, as chapter 7 described. There are possible solutions to these problems, ways to use these systems that would at least ameliorate the problems I have described. First, in contrast to the tendency toward the ever-greater minimization of risk, these systems could be used to limit screening and prescribing to merely the highest-risk groups. Polygenic risk scores create stratified risk groups, indicating low-, normal-, and high-risk patients for a condition. One could use these risk scores to identify and treat only high- or very high-risk patients, thus limiting risk reduction to those who will probably receive the greatest benefit.[17] Some scholars recommend this course of action, but many articles describe how to use PRSs or AI systems to move ever more people into screening and medication—in other words, to discover previously unknown risk groups, rather than to limit the numbers of people seen as at risk. Even in some studies that do try to limit the number of patients exposed to risk-reducing interventions, patients themselves reject being treated as low risk, preferring to do everything possible against any risk.[18]

Second, risk should be calculated only for a limited number of conditions for which there are highly effective interventions. This is a classic criterion for genetic testing, which is a sort of risk testing: you should do it only when the test is highly predictive and can lead to effective action. This tendency is being lost in the face of DTC testing and broader genomic screening. As one tests for risks of more conditions, there is a greater chance that an acknowledgment of risk will merely lead to worry or overtreatment.

Third, risk predictions need to be uncoupled from the sanctions for practitioners described in chapter 7, such as changes to reimbursement rates. Studies of the managerial use of metrics show that a blind faith in numbers will eventually lead to a less effective workforce, whose members ignore or lose their capabilities for prudential judgment or do absurd things merely to meet their metrics. Quality metrics like adherence to prescription guidelines work best when they are merely supplied to professionals without further threat of sanctions.[19] The professionals can then use the information to inform their prudential judgment. If they are below average at prescribing a risk-reducing medication, they can decide whether that is due to a problem in their current practice, a singularity of their patient population, or an explicit informed decision. When used in these ways, quality metrics can support rather than undermine prudence.

Finally, in line with supporting prudential judgment, AI systems should provide more rather than less information: a range of predictions, estimates of uncertainty, and the weight of different factors in coming to the prediction. Users need to know how systems come to decisions and what vulnerabilities they have. In general, practitioners should be trained to detect the limitations of any system they use. These features allow for greater prudence in judgment; users can assess and challenge reasons for a decision. Such explainability, however, might make these systems less powerful, would be difficult to implement, and would require changes in medical training.[20]

From Moonshot to Groundshot

Even if risk-based prevention and precision medicine have a positive role to play in the clinic, policymakers still need to determine how much of society's resources should be devoted to developing and implementing them. This question is especially salient in a world in which hundreds of millions of people lack access to effective treatments for serious infectious diseases. Is it just to spend billions of dollars for marginal gains in life expectancy among the world's wealthiest nations through risk reduction when there are easy ways to save many more young lives with that money? I doubt it. That is not to say that some research should not be done on this front, as one never knows where a breakthrough will occur that will help everyone. However, our investment in precision medicine is clearly out of proportion to its possible global benefits and the urgency of the problems it addresses.

To take the example of oncology, in 2016, the Obama administration funded a Cancer Moonshot championed by Vice President Biden that cost $1.6 billion.[21] In 2022, the Biden administration proposed another round of funding for Moonshot efforts. These funds contribute to the kind of precision medicine research discussed in this chapter. People hope that it might succeed where the War on Cancer of the 1970s failed.

Yet soon after the 2016 Cancer Moonshot was proposed, several oncologists noted that there were much easier and more direct ways to reduce deaths from cancer. Most cancer patients in the world, especially those in low- and middle-income countries, lack access to basic, proven, effective treatments. Fewer than 25 percent of cancer patients can access needed surgery for cancer.[22] The statistics are similarly dismal for radiation therapy, with more than 90 percent of patients in low-income countries going without necessary treatment.[23] These effective treatments need to become available in a consistent manner. Instead of a Cancer Moonshot, critical oncologists proposed a Groundshot: "This strategy would focus on the implementation of treatments that are already known to work, incentivising research on affordable and cost-effective interventions for cancer control, and strategies that can be applied globally to reduce cancer morbidity and mortality."[24] These oncologists are correct that we should be spending far more of our resources distributing highly effective treatments rather than developing what will probably be marginally effective ones.

Thus there is a role for these tools of risk reduction and genomics in the clinic, but it is probably limited. Even when used, they must be kept in check because of the tendency of actuarial bureaucracies to constantly expand the goals of risk reduction to the detriment of good medical care. Yet there will always remain the problem of high-risk patients who will not adjust their regimen or will not respond to risk reduction. In today's system of control, they tend to be eliminated or excluded. The last chapter will discuss how to ethically address these groups.

FOURTEEN

Institutions for Slow Medicine

Mercy House is a home for children run by a Franciscan order of Ugandan nuns.[1] At least, it describes itself as a home for children. Really, it takes in all kinds of people: orphans, children of the very poor, people with disabilities, older adults who have no family. The sisters take in pretty much anyone they encounter who is in need because they fall outside of Uganda's local systems of familial care and patronage or whose needs are too great for those systems. This ready response to need certainly does not help the home's meager budget. The sisters are constantly overstretched, and the grounds, food, and items provided to residents are certainly not luxurious. But the sisters facilitate decent care for the residents on the shoestring budget that always is threatening to break. People with diseases receive surgeries and medication; children go to school; everyone is fed. Moreover, they live in a community in which everyone participates. Children work in the garden plots, as they would if they lived with a family. Older kids in the dormitory look after the younger. They pray and play together. The care is fairly effective; many people with disabilities receive vocational training and rehabilitative care that allow them to eventually live independently. Children graduate from secondary school, and some even go to university. And those whose disabilities are too severe for independent living continue to be a valued part of the home. These are major accomplishments for an underfunded institution facing great need.

Despite this effectiveness in addressing significant challenges, over the last twenty-five years Mercy House has kept running into crises with its funders. The home had a few long-term funders among foundations, but as a younger generation educated in aid management replaced an earlier generation of charitable workers, the funders became hostile to Mercy House's methods: the home's business practices are not up-to-date; the House has little infrastructure for monitoring and evaluation; their approach is not sustainable, in the sense of financially stable. Funders wanted them to be more focused and efficient. A crisis occurred when an international organization providing aid for people with disabilities demanded that the sisters kick out all nondisabled residents so that they could more effectively focus care on those with disabilities. The sisters rejected casting out the aged, the poor, and orphans from the home. They knew their care was not optimized, but it was hard to see how it could be for many of their residents. Other threats came from the state, which, under pressure from international organizations, developed regulations that were intended to drive people out of institutional care because of its risks. The problem is that there is nowhere else for many of the residents to go and the home lacked the money to meet many of the Western-style regulations.[2] All of these measures gradually diminished Mercy House's ability to care, even though the measures were driven by demands to raise quality, increase safety, and reduce risks. Those people forced from Mercy House or who never made it there in the first place fall outside of the bureaucratic gaze, so their suffering is less of a problem to the state. Mercy House does not fit current paradigms of international aid because it does not optimize its population metrics. As China Scherz describes, it does not promise to end poverty or risk; it just cares for people in need.

As we have seen in earlier chapters, the aim of a population focus is to optimize: to have the best metrics, the most efficient procedures, the lowest risk. Yet as chapter 9 described, there remains the problem of people whose risks and suffering cannot be controlled, who face the threat of elimination or abandonment. The ideal in contemporary Western society is for everyone to receive care in the home from their family or a paid caregiver. It is an ideal we have foisted on other nations around the world. However, little is done for those without a family or whose family does not have appropriate resources or whose problems, such as mental illness or drug addiction, make living at home difficult. They are too often abandoned to the streets, where at least they do not show up in any institution's metrics.

Yet institutions like hospitals were founded exactly for those without family. Hospital-like care first arose in monastic communities in the fourth century.[3] Since the monks had renounced family support, large monastic communities had to find ways to provide care to the sick and infirm who otherwise would have received care from their families. To meet this demand, monasteries founded infirmaries that provided medical care, better food, and a place to rest or recuperate. By the end of the fourth century, monks were opening versions of these charitable institutions to others in society who lacked family or whose family could not care for them: migrants, the elderly, the sick, the very poor. Mercy House echoed the work of these early hospitals. These hospitals were not optimized or risk reducing. They filled in gaps to care for those in need who had been excluded from surrounding society. Today, though, institutions that serve these purposes often are undermined by demands for optimization and a demand for scalability. This chapter argues that we still need such institutions for those who fall outside the logic of risk reduction and the kind of medicine such a logic can offer.

Slow Medicine

Mercy House is one example of such an institution, but there are others in the recent past, such as Laguna Honda Hospital in San Francisco, as described by Victoria Sweet,[4] a doctor trained in the history of medicine. At the hospital, she worked with extremely sick people with chronic illnesses or with disabilities that were difficult to address. Many of her patients suffered from broader problems such as substance abuse, homelessness, and histories of trauma. These patients needed too much time and attention to be cost-effective to treat in a regular hospital, so they were sent to Laguna Honda, which served as a safety net for the city. Even at Laguna Honda, they would be discharged for their immediate medical needs, only to frequently get sick again, returning for readmission. These were the high-cost patients that efficient value-based care tries to address.

Over her many years at Laguna Honda, Sweet developed the skills required for caring for these complex patients. She found that what they needed was not intensive testing (although certain tests could provide helpful information) or genomics or a risk score. They needed the careful attention that it takes to provide a good diagnosis. The doctor needed to take time to get to the root of the problem. She argues for the importance of the careful physical examination, which is all too often forgone in today's clinics because of time constraints. Moreover, the patients needed time for healing to occur. Sweet prescribed treatments, of course, but, drawing on her studies of medieval medicine, she ultimately thought these medications just provided an aid to the patient's own powers of healing. In the premodern vision, nature heals itself.

This framework inspired Sweet to propose what she calls a slow medicine that would replace our fast, high-intervention, risky medicine. Others have called it a gentle medicine because it is much more hesitant to intervene with pharmaceuticals, surgeries, and other procedures than is precision medicine or even standard curative medicine.[5] This form of medicine is more likely to encourage the doctor to watch and wait, giving her the time to perform a careful examination and take a medical history, because it is built on the classic doctor-patient relationship. For those patients at the highest risk, with the most serious problems, this kind of slow medicine can do wonders, as Sweet describes. This medicine focuses on care.[6]

To succeed, slow medicine needs institutions that will support it. Laguna Honda was one such institution. Its open wards allowed community to form among patients and an easy accessibility of patients to doctors and nurses. Its beautiful setting promoted healing. Most of all it simply allowed people time to heal. It was not the revolving door of many recovery hospitals in which patients are sent home, have a scary moment or a dramatic change of condition, go to the emergency room, stay in the hospital briefly, are sent to a recovery center for longer, and then are sent home again, with the cycle repeating over and over again.[7] Instead, Laguna Honda allowed them to stay for as long as needed.

This kind of institution is unintelligible to modern accountants, risk analysts, and policymakers.[8] It is not optimized. It cannot describe exactly its timeline or metrics for success. To others, it may even seem like a rights violation, as patients are not being cared for in a home, even if they do not have any homes. Thus lawyers, activists, and city health officials all conspired to destroy the old Laguna Honda and bring a more efficient, optimized institution into being.

Similarly, U.S. hospice was originally designed to allow terminally ill patients to die in hospice institutions, provided with specialized medical care and continuous support. That proved expensive, though, so hospice organizations and the legislation that funds them depend on family caregivers, assisted by occasional visits by hospice staff. There is little support available for those without family or whose families lack the skill or time to care for them at home through a long dying process.[9]

Such contemporary optimized institutions will not allow the same space and time for healing to occur. That is why we need to make room for institutions that allow for slow medicine. These institutions would make time, allow staff to be with the patients. They would not worry about optimization. They would provide a space for those whose risks cannot be controlled and who otherwise would be relegated to homelessness, prison, or death. Institutions like this do continue to exist: Laguna Honda or Mercy House. They are under pressure, though, from the expanding logic of risk reduction.

Reducing Cost and Risk

Since the 1960s, many forms of institutional care have been dramatically scaled back. Long-term care hospitals are under dramatic pressure from funders to get patients home. The size of mental asylums was drastically reduced after the deinstitutionalization movement. Orphanages have been replaced by foster care. The reasons for these shifts are complex, but they in part arise from good intentions to reduce cost and risk, although it is unclear that these shifts have succeeded in their goals.

First, it is expensive to run these kinds of institutions, especially if there is no clear plan for decreasing the patient population over the long run. Institutions demand long-term, consistent funding. In contrast, contemporary funders want solutions that will make problems eventually disappear. They want the end of poverty.[10] Large institutions of the kind described above, however, assume that the poor will always be with us.[11] Their existence asserts a future of continued need. Progress will not cause the problems of homelessness, substance abuse, or mental illness to vanish.

The solidity of institutions symbolizes the permanence of these problems and makes a claim for continued funding. Any progress on these problems largely occurs at the level of the individual, and these successes are achieved only slowly at best. Institutions for slow medicine thus exist as an affront to some of our basic political myths: progress, the perfect solution, and cost control.

Yet one might ask how costly such institutions would be compared to alternatives. High-cost patients consume large amounts of medical spending already, and risk-based, targeted programs have proven ineffective in randomized controlled trials.[12] Prison, where many people with mental illness end up, is certainly expensive, as is in-home care. As Sweet narrates in many of her cases, while Laguna Honda's investment in patients was initially substantial, the healing that occurred may have been more cost-effective than other strategies.[13] Unless massive, randomized controlled trials are run, the question of cost is open.

There are also clear risks of abuse in institutions. One need only read the harrowing narratives of Ireland's Magdalen laundries, Dickens's literary descriptions of Victorian orphanages and workhouses, or critiques of mental institutions to realize the extent of physical and mental violence that can be inflicted on inmates in such institutions.[14] Such institutions can simply become a zone of exclusion imposed by society on those who do not conform.[15] Further, there are more subtle questions raised by social scientists of what kind of discipline is being enforced and whether it undermines the inmates' autonomy.[16] Institutions can serve as powerful tools of social control or individual tyranny.

Even though these dangers can exist in healthcare institutions, we must also take note that many of the same problems bedevil their alternatives. Prison certainly contains the risk of violent abuse. Living on the streets can be a harrowing experience. Abuse occurs in families and in foster care. The second part of this book described the danger of manipulation or abandonment in risk-based public health. Optimization leads to its own dangers. In fact, all social forms, all mechanisms that rely on power, contain dangers. The question is what balance of opportunities versus dangers exist in each social arrangement and which framework strives for better values. In this case, I would suggest further exploration of institutions for slow medicine.

Scalability

One of the ways that the institutions I have described try to protect against such dangers is that their workers are motivated by more than the purely bureaucratic ends of the institutions or a paycheck. The doctors and nurses of Laguna Honda, even the support staff, are animated by older ideals of the healing relationship. Sweet describes how some new staff just did not fit, in part because their values were not aligned with the institution's. Mercy House worked as well as it did because the sisters were animated by a charity inspired by Christianity. Not every sister fit. There were some who, by their own admission, lacked the heart for helping, even though they might want to develop it.[17] These sisters did not provide the kind of care necessary, and most everyone recognized this fact. Such institutions thus require a very particular kind of staff animated by concern for those who are at high risk.

The need for staff who possess certain virtues creates another objection to institutions for slow medicine. They are not scalable in the same way that risk-reducing medical programs are. For high-cost patient programs, all you need is the algorithm and staff with defined technical roles. Wellness programs can be endlessly scaled up through an internet portal and by hiring a couple more wellness coaches. 23andMe can scan the genomes of everyone. Anonymous statistical care is easy to replicate by any person or program.

Institutions of slow medicine are not like that. They require practitioners with certain dispositions. Only certain people have these virtues, or they require a long training to form. Thus these institutions can be undermined through attempts to scale them up. More and more workers might be brought in too quickly to properly shape their dispositions. In such cases, the institution either becomes ineffective or must start operating like an optimized institution. They are thus fragile things.

Even authors who recognize the value of care in institutional settings can despair of them as a solution to our problems for reasons of scalability. For example, Harold Braswell's ethnography of hospice demonstrates the failings of our hospice system because it depends on family caregivers.[18] There are too many people who lack a family able to provide care, who thus face a difficult death. In his study, some of these patients found a solution to their lack of family caregivers in a hospice run by a group of Catholic nuns that provided long-term institutional care for free. The care is, by all reports, outstanding: personal, compassionate, technically competent, and spiritually rich. The nuns are able to provide good care only because they fall outside of the insurance system, depending on charitable donations rather than reimbursements from companies or government programs. Despite his admiration for the sisters, Braswell ultimately dismisses them as a response to the problem of hospice because of the difficulty of scaling up their work to the whole nation. The sisters' care is founded in a specific religious motivation of Christian charity. In responding to the dying patient, they seek to respond to the dying Christ on the cross. This response is solidified in virtues built through a lifetime of prayer, meditation, worship, and other devotional practices. This kind of formation is not scalable, at least not in a secular society.[19] The answer might be to not try to scale this kind of care. Maybe the care required for slow medicine can only emerge at the local level in the desire to accompany the suffering other. Efforts of care may not solve a problem for all of society, but they may at least address the suffering immediately in front of the caregiver.

Perhaps, though, these institutions' failure to scale is not anomalous. Even programs designed to be scalable do not necessarily succeed in their expansion. For example, a report in the scientific journal *Nature* detailed the benefits but also the problems of using randomized controlled trials to analyze the effectiveness of international programs addressing poverty and health. Many programs that succeed in their initial small-scale trials become less successful as they expand. One researcher working on a project that engaged mothers in order to improve child development found that her program, while very successful in its initial small trial in Jamaica, did not have as significant an effect when expanded in Colombia and Peru. She took the lesson as being that "scaling up interventions that depend on complex human interactions won't be easy" because "people are going in and building relationships and helping parents become better parents. That is more difficult" than something like a cash-transfer program.[20] Even programs that may seem to eschew a demand for virtue actually require it.

Concluding Thoughts

Certain institutional forms are able to provide good care for those who are in danger of being abandoned or eliminated by risk-based medicine. They allow the time for slow medicine and genuine care for the patient. Yet they run against many contemporary social values, such as cost-effectiveness, auditability, autonomy, and scalability. They contain risks of abuse. Moreover, they require certain kinds of people as staff. For these reasons, they are not an easy policy solution. Yet they may be the best way to care for those who might otherwise be abandoned. These are not institutions that can be easily started through policy initiatives, so my plea on their behalf is relatively modest: governments and policymakers should at least try to make room for their survival, rather than destroying them through attempts at optimization.

This need to ensure the space for virtues like charity to function is just one aspect of a broader need to protect the virtues of medicine from the optimizing trend of risk assessment. We need to create clinics that protect the clinical judgment of the medical practitioner, allowing her to not press risk-based tests or medication on patients for whom she judges they are not appropriate. We need to aid the prudence, temperance, and courage of patients, allowing them to enjoy their good health without anxiety or a desperate attempt to extend life. Such spaces can exist only if we set limits to prevention and accept that as finite beings we must accept risks, and ultimately mortality, if we want to flourish in the present.

NOTES

PREFACE

1. Collins, *Language of Life*, xxiv.
2. For overviews of virtue ethics, see Aristotle, *Nicomachean Ethics*; MacIntyre, *After Virtue*; Annas, *Morality of Happiness*; Hursthouse, *On Virtue Ethics*; Cloutier and Mattison III, "Resurgence of Virtue."
3. For an example of comparative virtue ethics, see Yearley, *Mencius and Aquinas*.
4. Pellegrino and Thomasma, *Virtues in Medical Practice*; Pellegrino and Thomasma, *Christian Virtues*.

CHAPTER ONE   Suspicion of the Body

1. N. Price et al., "Wellness Study"; Cross, "'Scientific Wellness' Study."
2. This is the traditional definition of the aim of medicine at least since the time of Plato (*Euthydemus* 291e). There are alternative understandings such as to reduce suffering (Cassell, *Nature of Suffering*), to respond to autonomous patient demands, or to achieve the patient's good (Pellegrino and Thomasma, *For the Patient's Good*), but health still seems to be the best framework in which to analyze the goals of medicine. For critique of other aims of medicine, such as the reduction of suffering, see Curlin, "Hospice."
3. There is a vast literature on the meaning of health. For helpful overviews of the debates over health, see Svenaeus, *Hermeneutics of Medicine*, 59–83; Messer, *Flourishing*, 1–50. The phenomenological definition provided by Svenaeus will serve as my major guide in this chapter. His, and in turn my, understanding draws on a large body of previous works on the phenomenology of health, such as Pellegrino and Thomasma, *Philosophical Basis*; Canguilhem, *Normal and the Pathological*; Leder, *Absent Body*; Toombs, *Meaning of Illness*; Gadamer, *Enigma of Health*. For

contrasting understandings, such as the biostatistical or holistic models, see Boorse, "Health"; Nordenfelt, *On the Nature of Health*. Later chapters will also engage the World Health Organization's definition of health and criticisms of it. In this book, I am restricting my analysis to physical health. Mental health and the definition of mental illness raise a number of distinct concerns that are frequently unrelated to the ones I address here.

4. Canguilhem, *Normal and the Pathological*, 91.

5. Gadamer, *Enigma of Health*, 112.

6. See discussions in Nutton, *Ancient Medicine*; Klibansky, Panofsky, and Saxl, *Saturn and Melancholy*. There was a correspondence between medical health and moral virtue: health is the rational balance of the body, just as virtue is a rational mean of the dispositions. Virtue and health reflect harmonious dispositions, whereas disease and vice are imbalance.

7. Svenaeus, *Hermeneutics of Medicine*, 93.

8. This is a particular theme of Leder, *Absent Body*. Other experiences also can draw attention to the body, such as intense pleasure or exertion.

9. See Aristotle, *On the Soul* 2.1.

10. For these phenomenological discussions of tools, see Heidegger, *Being and Time*, 98–99; Polanyi, *Personal Knowledge*, 59; Crawford, *World beyond Your Head*.

11. Heidegger, *Being and Time*, 102–7.

12. Leder, *Absent Body*; Svenaeus, *Hermeneutics of Medicine*, 106–13.

13. For more on this alterity of the body, see the discussion below of McKenny, *To Relieve the Human Condition*.

14. For the rhythmic nature of life as discussed in these paragraphs, see Svenaeus, *Hermeneutics of Medicine*, 94–100.

15. Ivan Illich, in *Limits to Medicine*, 63, describes how medicine has removed much of the common pharmacopeia of preindustrial societies but has also added to it.

16. For a discussion of the importance of accepting these limitations and a description of the powerful forces in our culture that push against that acceptance, see Davis and Scherz, *Evening of Life*.

17. This is the problem of transhumanism. Transhumanists refuse to be at home in the body and see its limitations only as things to overcome. For discussions of transhumanism, see McKenny, *Biotechnology, Human Nature*; Cole-Turner, *Transhumanism and Transcendence*; Bostrom, "Why I Want to Be a Posthuman."

18. Georges Canguilhem is the primary source for this model of health and disease; see Canguilhem, *Normal and the Pathological*. See also Gadamer, *Enigma of Health*.

19. Debates over disability, health, and normality are complex, and I will not be dealing with them in any depth here. For discussion, see Barnes, *Minority Body*;

Messer, *Flourishing*; Toombs, *Meaning of Illness*; Romero, "Disability, Catholic Questions"; Berkman and Boeré, "St. Thomas Aquinas on Impairment."

20. For the importance of coping in discussions of everyday pain and discomfort, see Hadler, *Worried Sick*.

21. This discussion draws on the picture of the healing relationship described by Pellegrino and Thomasma, *Philosophical Basis*; Cassell, *Nature of Suffering*. As many have noted, it is dangerous to view medicine as aimed only at the relief of suffering, as this can lead to extreme measures to destroy the sufferer. See Hauerwas, *Suffering Presence*; Curlin, "Hospice." While recognizing these dangers, it is still important to note that suffering sets the context that calls forth the clinical encounter.

22. Pellegrino and Thomasma, *Virtues in Medical Practice*; Pellegrino and Thomasma, *Christian Virtues*.

23. For a similar disclaimer, see Hadler, *Last Well Person*.

24. Preventive forms of medicine are not the only social phenomenon that alienates us from our bodies. Many people, especially women, feel dissatisfaction with their bodily appearance and performance, contributing to pathologies like depression or eating disorders. This dissatisfaction is inspired by dangerous social ideals instead of health, so it is different from what is discussed here. There are overlaps with aspects of my argument here, though, in that dissatisfaction is in part driven by quantitative objectification of the body through measures like weight, and it is accentuated by technologies like social media that encourage comparison with ideal others. Experiences of difference or prejudice, like racism, can make a person feel alienated from the body. Again, this alienation results from problematic social encounters and so is different from my discussion, unless the alienation becomes somaticized, as it often does, in which case it collapses into my general understanding of disease.

25. The next chapter will trace the development of risk-based medicine. My primary sources for this phenomenon are Aronowitz, *Risky Medicine*; Dumit, *Drugs for Life*; Welch, Schwartz, and Woloshin, *Overdiagnosed*; Greene, *Prescribing by Numbers*; Hadler, *Last Well Person*. See also Illich, *Limits to Medicine*, 89–97.

26. For descriptions of these experiences, see Dumit, *Drugs for Life*, chap. 1; Löwy, *Preventive Strikes*; Svenaeus, *Hermeneutics of Medicine*, 104–6; Aronowitz, *Unnatural History*; Ehrenreich, *Natural Causes*, 5.

27. Gillespie, "Experience of Risk."

28. For an overview of the Quantified Self movement, see Droge, "What Is Quantified Self?"; Lupton, *Quantified Self*; Schull, "Data for Life"; Schull, "Data-Based Self."

29. Ioannidis et al., "How to Survive."

30. Another bodily state that does not quite fit the framework I develop in this chapter is pregnancy. It is a natural condition experienced by the majority of women

across history. To think of it as a disease experience is incorrect, as feminist critics of the medicalization of pregnancy have noted. Yet it also raises particular dangers and is unfamiliar to the first-time mother, so it does require preventive care. Too much prevention, though, leads to care strategies like twilight sleep or elevated rates of Caesarean sections. The re-embrace of midwifery as a practice separate from though allied to medicine suggests that pregnancy is different from standard health complaints and thus requires, as a first response, a different kind of profession that ideally is alive to risk but not in a medicalized way.

31. "Prevent, v."

32. Ps 119:148. Compare the NRSV translation: "My eyes are awake before each watch of the night, that I may meditate on your promise."

33. Rom 7:23–24. Gerald McKenny describes this Pauline vision of the body in relation to phenomenological discussions of health and disease in McKenny, *To Relieve the Human Condition*, 211–26. This of course is not the only Christian understanding of the body, as other important sources indicate; see Brown, *Body and Society*; Bynum, *Fragmentation and Redemption*; John Paul II, *Man and Woman*.

34. For a discussion of how ancient ascetic practices of the self that transformed desire were adopted by early Christianity, see Hadot, *Philosophy*; Foucault, *Hermeneutics of the Subject*; P. Scherz, *Science and Christian Ethics*.

35. 2 Cor 5:4. As this verse indicates, bodily resurrection is extremely important for Christian (as well as other Abrahamic religions') understandings of health, risk, and death. My focus in this book will largely be on the ways a focus on risk disrupts temporal flourishing rather than on the ways that it distracts Christians from trust in God and hope in eternal life, as important as those effects are. For reflections on medical risk with regard to larger Christian themes and through the lens of scripture, see Curlin, "'Sufficient for the Day'"; Kavin Rowe, "Theology, Medicalization, and Risk"; Gregory, "Tree of Life."

36. Admittedly, recent research shows that Gnosticism was a complex phenomenon, comprising a diverse set of groups with different aims and orientations for which we have little direct evidence. Our understanding mostly comes from the Gnostics' Orthodox opponents. Here, my goal is to describe a Gnostic tendency as reconstructed by the church fathers, such as Irenaeus, Tertullian, and Augustine, and modern scholars such as Jonas, *Gnostic Religion*. I also draw on the depiction of Gnosticism in recent Catholic documents, especially those released under Pope Francis: "[Gnosticism] presumes to liberate the human person from the body and from the material universe, in which traces of the provident hand of the Creator are no longer found, but only a reality deprived of meaning, foreign to the fundamental identity of the person, and easily manipulated by the interests of man" (Congregation for the Doctrine of the Faith, "Placuit Deo").

37. E.g., Waters, *This Mortal Flesh*; McKenny, *To Relieve the Human Condition*, 220–22.

38. In this way, it is similar to twentieth-century existentialism as described by Jonas, *Gnostic Religion*, 320–40. Humans are alienated from the world with no possibility for salvation.

39. For cancer survivors' ongoing experience of risk and anxiety, see Aronowitz, *Risky Medicine*, 137–56; Löwy, *Preventive Strikes*.

40. As these chapters will describe, neither the knowledge claims nor the technical effectiveness of the medicine of risk control is quite as firm as proponents of precision medicine claim.

CHAPTER TWO   Sicken to Shun Sickness

1. For a discussion of earlier modes of medicine, see Starr, *Social Transformation*. Insurance companies drove the rise of yearly checkups as a way to control life insurance costs. See Bouk, *How Our Days Became Numbered*.

2. For a history of the reduction of deaths from infectious diseases, see McKeown, *Modern Rise of Population*.

3. Centers for Disease Control, "Leading Causes of Death."

4. Centers for Disease Control, "Faststats."

5. This was untrue. As with most health conditions, cardiovascular disease can also strike down poor workers at younger ages. Michael Marmot has explored the effects of social status on life expectancy, showing that lower-status groups almost always have worse outcomes, including for cardiovascular disease. His theory, which chapter 11 will explore in more depth, is that the stress of low social status is worse than the stress of a difficult job in which you at least have some control. See Marmot, *Status Syndrome*; Marmot, *Health Gap*.

6. Enos, Beyer, and Holmes, "Pathogenesis of Coronary Disease." For a discussion of this study in light of other research on risk factors for heart disease, see Greene, *Prescribing by Numbers*, 157.

7. For the Framingham Study's history and impact, see Aronowitz, *Risky Medicine*, 69–93; Dumit, *Drugs for Life*, 114–17.

8. Greene, *Prescribing by Numbers*, 7.

9. For example, Greene, *Prescribing by Numbers*; Dumit, *Drugs for Life*.

10. For history, see Greene, *Prescribing by Numbers*, 21–50.

11. Greene, *Prescribing by Numbers*, 151–88.

12. Quoted in Greene, *Prescribing by Numbers*, 2. See similar discussion of how treatments that restore health limit corporate profitability in Dumit, *Drugs for Life*, 177ff.

13. Dumit, *Drugs for Life*, 152–54.

14. Centers for Disease Control, "Leading Causes of Death"; Centers for Disease Control, "Faststats."

15. Aronowitz, *Unnatural History*, 144–47; Löwy, *Preventive Strikes*, 119ff.

16. Löwy, *Preventive Strikes*, 88; Aronowitz, *Unnatural History*, 161, 178–81.

17. Aronowitz, *Unnatural History*, 218–21; Löwy, *Preventive Strikes*, 145.

18. Aronowitz, *Unnatural History*, 225–34; Löwy, *Preventive Strikes*, 145–49.

19. The list of critics is broad, but my discussion draws especially on Hadler, *Last Well Person*; Greene, *Prescribing by Numbers*; Löwy, *Preventive Strikes*; Welch, Schwartz, and Woloshin, *Overdiagnosed*; Dumit, *Drugs for Life*; Aronowitz, *Unnatural History*; Aronowitz, *Risky Medicine*; Stegenga, *Medical Nihilism*. Some medical journals have also begun to question overtreatment and overdiagnosis, as seen in features such as *JAMA Internal Medicine*'s "Less Is More" and the *British Medical Journal*'s "Too Much Medicine" initiatives.

20. For a (perhaps overly) broad critique of iatrogenic disease, see Illich, *Limits to Medicine*.

21. For a history of these debates over the relative risks and benefits of mammography, especially for women under age fifty, see Aronowitz, *Unnatural History*, 235–55.

22. For a thorough discussion of the difficulties of the expert patient in negotiating how to respond to a PSA test, see Dumit, *Drugs for Life*, 27–54. The procedure is becoming less common because of many criticisms, but it is still available.

23. The U.K.'s regulatory body has recommended that patients first have an MRI of the prostate to detect cancer rather than beginning with a biopsy. National Institute for Health and Care Excellence, "Prostate Cancer."

24. U.S. Preventive Services Task Force, "Final Recommendation Statement."

25. For a discussion of the anxiety of choosing between multiple future possibilities, see P. Scherz, *Tomorrow's Troubles*, 31–59.

26. A metanalysis of available clinical trial data for statins suggested no significant side effects (U.S. Preventive Services Task Force, "Statin Use"). However, individual trials have reported side effects, like increased rates of diabetes and muscle problems, among those on statins, as have observational reports (Redberg and Katz, "Statins for Primary Prevention"; Thompson et al., "Statin-Associated Side Effects"). The reasons for these discrepancies are unclear. People suspicious of the use of statins in primary prevention point to the generally younger groups of patients used in trials and the industry control over most trials.

27. National Center for Health Statistics, *Health, United States, 2016*.

28. Bretthauer et al., "Effect of Colonoscopy Screening." This study has been criticized because only 42 percent of people invited for screening colonoscopies actually received them. That probably reflects real-world rates of uptake, so it is an

accurate pragmatic trial of the screening problem (Mandrola and Prasad, "Screening Colonoscopy"). Even so, the authors performed a statistical analysis to examine the efficacy only among those who actually received the colonoscopy, which introduces confounding effects (i.e., people who choose a colonoscopy are probably more health conscious in general). Even with just these people, though, colonoscopies reduced all-cause mortality by only .15 percent over ten years (giving a 10.88 percent rather than an 11.03 percent chance of death). It is unclear that such an improvement is worth the trouble.

29. U.S. Preventive Services Task Force, "Statin Use," 746.

30. U.S. Preventive Services Task Force, "Statin Use," 756; Habib, Katz, and Redberg, "Statins."

31. Krogsbøll, Jørgensen, and Gøtzsche, "General Health Checks."

32. As Dumit describes in *Drugs for Life*, 117, clinical trials now "correlate mass population treatments with statistical population health improvement."

33. Aronowitz, *Unnatural History*, 171–78.

34. Jahn, Giovannucci, and Stampfer, "High Prevalence." Similar studies have found a widespread prevalence of breast cancers and thyroid cancers in autopsies, with "virtually all people aged 50 to 70" carrying in situ thyroid cancers. See discussion and notes in Löwy, *Preventive Strikes*, 151.

35. U.S. Preventive Services Task Force, "Statin Use," 756.

36. Dumit, *Drugs for Life*, 151–55. For a similar critique of the clinical trial system, see Kaufman, *Ordinary Medicine*.

37. Lundh et al., "Industry Sponsorship."

CHAPTER THREE   Genetics and Risk

1. Regalado, "World's First Gattaca Baby Tests"; P. Scherz, "Life as an Intelligence Test." For more information on their offerings, see the company's website, www.lifeview.com/lifeview.

2. See the remarks at the ceremony marking the supposed completion of the Human Genome Project, Clinton et al., "Reading the Book of Life"; Collins, *Language of Life*. For a seminal analysis of the problem with these descriptions, see Nelkin and Lindee, *DNA Mystique*.

3. This historical narrative draws on Porter, *Rise of Statistical Thinking*; Ewald, *État Providence*; Hacking, *Taming of Chance*; Desrosieres, *Politics of Large Numbers*; Bernstein, *Against the Gods*. For ethical analysis, see P. Scherz, *Tomorrow's Troubles*, 93–116; P. Scherz, "No Acceptable Losses."

4. Foucault, *Security, Territory, Population*. There is another large contributor to the rise of a focus on risk and population: the insurance industry. The

nineteenth century saw the professionalization of actuarial science. By examining different cohorts, life insurance companies started to dissect the risk factors leading to differential life expectancy. Initially, this information was used only to adjust insurance premiums or disqualify applicants, but eventually it began to be used in campaigns of prevention. For a history of these preventive efforts, see Bouk, *How Our Days Became Numbered*. Life insurance companies were the first ones to advise people to have yearly checkups with nurses and even inspired manuals for healthy living, like Fisher and Fisk, *How to Live*. In the early twentieth century, most of the advice was about lifestyle (e.g., lose weight, get fresh air) of the sort I will discuss in chapter 12. By the time health insurance companies started to embrace the kinds of preventive care discussed in the last chapter, these preventive measures had already become paradigmatic in medicine.

Another contributor to the development of a population focus was workers' compensation insurance, as discussed in Ewald, *État Providence*; Witt, *Accidental Republic*. For a broader discussion and analysis of these trends, see P. Scherz, *Tomorrow's Troubles*, 93–116.

5. For history of the critical role of asylums in the rise of eugenics, see Porter, *Genetics in the Madhouse*. Asylums were also key to the development of programs of Nazi euthanasia and to later forms of unethical medical research, as discussed in Burleigh, *Death and Deliverance*; Rothman, *Strangers at the Bedside*.

6. On the tie between eugenics and the professional middle class, see MacKenzie, *Statistics in Britain*, 15–50.

7. The literature on the history of eugenics is vast, but for some helpful overviews of aspects of that movement, see MacKenzie, *Statistics in Britain*; Kevles, *In the Name of Eugenics*; Paul, *Politics of Heredity*; Carlson, *Unfit*; Porter, *Karl Pearson*; Müller-Wille and Rheinberger, *Cultural History of Heredity*.

8. Though historical focus has rightly been on these horrible aspects of the eugenics movement, eugenics was quite diverse and led in many policy directions, sometimes coinciding with other reformist health movements of the time. For example, many eugenicists argued for supporting large families to the point that they gained support from religious figures otherwise opposed to their other policy goals like sterilization laws. For the story of American Catholic engagement with the eugenic movement along these lines, see Leon, *Image of God*; Pavuk, *Respectably Catholic and Scientific*.

9. Müller-Wille and Rheinberger, *Cultural History of Heredity*, 6; Olby, *Origins of Mendelism*, 55–68.

10. For Pearson, see Porter, *Karl Pearson*.

11. For Pearson as institution-builder, see MacKenzie, *Statistics in Britain*, 94–119.

12. Porter, *Karl Pearson*, 285.
13. Müller-Wille and Rheinberger, *Cultural History of Heredity*, 2.
14. Porter, *Genetics in the Madhouse*, 242.
15. For history of the rise of Mendelian genetics, see Olby, *Origins of Mendelism*; Bowler, *Mendelian Revolution*. As these narratives reveal, the story of the rediscovery is not as simple as is commonly portrayed.
16. Popenoe, "Feeblemindedness."
17. For the history of scientific evidence and debate surrounding the category of feeble-mindedness, see Barker, "Biology of Stupidity"; Paul, *Politics of Heredity*, 117–32; Spencer and Paul, "Failure of a Scientific Critique."
18. For the history of this debate, see Provine, *Origins of Theoretical Population Genetics*, 56–89; MacKenzie and Barnes, "Scientific Judgment"; MacKenzie, *Statistics in Britain*, 120–52.
19. For this history, see Provine, *Origins of Theoretical Population Genetics*.
20. Some eugenicists were willing to countenance these approaches, even with these problems. See Paul, *Politics of Heredity*.
21. For discussion, see Stern, *Telling Genes*; Kevles, *In the Name of Eugenics*.
22. Population genetics was not wholly disconnected from social issues and fears of the unfit, though, with certain population geneticists and allied psychologists claiming that there were genetic distinctions between different racial groups and with sociobiologists arguing for biological roots to social problems. For an overview, see Panofsky, *Misbehaving Science*. Important works in this controversy include Jensen, "How Much Can We Boost I.Q."; Ann Arbor Science for the People Editorial Collective, *Biology as a Social Weapon*; Herrnstein and Murray, *Bell Curve*; Gould, *Mismeasure of Man*; Lewontin, *Biology as Ideology*.
23. Moreover, these theories have faced vigorous opposition from other scholars in evolutionary biology and population genetics. See, e.g., Coop et al., "Troublesome Inheritance," a letter written in response to Wade, *Troublesome Inheritance*.
24. Kay, *Molecular Vision of Life*.
25. For history, see Judson, *Eighth Day of Creation*.
26. Kay, *Molecular Vision of Life*, 195–98; Müller-Wille and Rheinberger, *Cultural History of Heredity*, 176.
27. Kay, *Who Wrote the Book of Life?*
28. However, even many genetic diseases are not straightforwardly deterministic. For a broader discussion of genetic variability and determinism, see chapter 4 and Alexander, *Genes, Determinism, and God*.
29. For discussion of this more liberal model of eugenics, see Savulescu, "Procreative Beneficence"; Agar, *Liberal Eugenics*.

30. The problematic assumptions about suffering and disability as well as the value of the lives of those with disability that this framework embraces have been ably explored and debunked by a vast number of works in disability studies. For a good overview, see Stahl, *Disability's Challenge to Theology*.

31. The possibilities of genetic engineering have led to a long debate about its eugenic overtones as well as numerous, contested frameworks to limit its applications, such as the therapy/enhancement distinction. For some of these discussions, see Ramsey, *Fabricated Man*; Kass, *Life, Liberty*; Harris, *Enhancing Evolution*; President's Council on Bioethics [U.S.], *Beyond Therapy*.

32. For background on CRISPR, see Lander, "Heroes of CRISPR"; Wright, Nuñez, and Doudna, "Biology and Applications"; P. Scherz, "Mechanism and Applications"; Doudna and Sternberg, *Crack in Creation*; Baylis, *Altered Inheritance*; Greely, *CRISPR People*.

33. Löwy, *Preventive Strikes*.

34. Zuboff, *Age of Surveillance Capitalism*; P. Scherz, *Tomorrow's Troubles*, 117–61.

35. Stevens, *Life Out of Sequence*; Reardon, *Postgenomic Condition*; P. Scherz, "Displacement of Human Judgment."

36. Schull, "Data for Life."

37. For defense and explanation of these methods, see Plomin, *Blueprint*; Harden, *Genetic Lottery*.

38. There is also a movement toward whole-genome sequencing, but that is at an early stage because of cost. For an early engagement with whole-genome sequencing, see Angrist, *Here Is a Human Being*. Otherwise, see the articles in the special supplement introduced by Johnston et al., "Sequencing Newborns."

39. For some of these critiques, see Sahlins, *Use and Abuse*; Nelkin and Lindee, *DNA Mystique*; McKinnon, *Neo-liberal Genetics*.

40. For the positivism and idealism that underlay Pearson's understanding of scientific investigation and contributed to his commitment to and framework for statistics, see Pearson, *Grammar of Science*; Porter, *Karl Pearson*. For a discussion of the contemporary positivism of the genetic research enterprise as it embraces the Big Data paradigms of genomics, see Allen, "Hypothesis, Induction"; Smalheiser, "Informatics"; Kell and Oliver, "Here Is the Evidence"; C. Anderson, "End of Theory"; P. Scherz, "Displacement of Human Judgment."

CHAPTER FOUR   Individuals and Populations

1. I draw the details of the BiDil story from Roberts, *Fatal Invention*, 168–89.

2. This argument was initially made in Lewontin, "Apportionment of Human Diversity." For further developments, see Roberts, *Fatal Invention*; Sussman, *Myth of Race*; Teslow, *Constructing Race*; Marks, *Is Science Racist?*

3. Bell, Kivimäki, and Batty, "Subgroup Analysis."

4. See discussion in P. Scherz, *Science and Christian Ethics*, chap. 1. For further discussions of the problems of statistics in research, see National Academies of Sciences, *Statistical Challenges*; Leek et al., "Five Ways to Fix Statistics"; Nuijten, "Practical Tools and Strategies"; Prasad, *Malignant*.

A similar debate surrounded the more recent FDA approval of an Alzheimer's drug, Aduhelm, which required a controversial reanalysis of the clinical trial results to find statistical significance. See Belluck, Kaplan, and Robbins, "How an Unproven Alzheimer's Drug Got Approved"; Servick, "Alzheimer's Drug Approved."

5. Krieger, "Who and What Is a 'Population'?"; Mathieson and Scally, "What Is Ancestry?"

6. Fortun, *Promising Genomics*.

7. Popejoy and Fullerton, "Genomics Is Failing"; Landry et al., "Lack of Diversity." There has been a recent growth in genomic analyses of Asian populations, largely because of research in industrialized Asian nations.

8. As an example of this shift, the group selected by the U.K. Biobank project in 2012–13 was 96 percent white (U.K. Biobank, "Repeat Assessment"). In contrast, in January 2023 the All of Us project reported a study population that is around 54 percent white, 21 percent black, and 17 percent Hispanic for whole-genome sequencing (All of Us, "Genomic Variants").

9. Mapes et al., "Diversity and Inclusion." It of course remains to be seen how successful this recruitment is.

10. Townes, *Breaking the Fine Rain of Death*; Skloot, *Immortal Life*.

11. For some of the positive engagements of racial minorities with genetics, see Nelson, *Social Life of DNA*.

12. This discussion draws on the analysis of these problems found in Kaplan and Fullerton, "Polygenic Risk."

13. James et al., "Limits of Personalization."

14. This inherent bias of all statistical samples has been a major problem for the algorithms developed by technology companies, which depend on statistical prediction.

15. Knight, *Risk, Uncertainty and Profit*.

16. Knight, *Risk, Uncertainty and Profit*, 234.

17. Childers, *Philosophy and Probability*.

18. Juengst et al., "From 'Personalized' to 'Precision' Medicine."

19. National Cancer Institute, "BRCA Gene Mutations."

20. Gould, "Median Isn't the Message."

CHAPTER FIVE   Public Health Ethics and Clinical Ethics

1. Rozier, "When Populations Become the Patient," 5. For similar retellings of parables, see Rozier, "Religion and Public Health," 1055; Rozier, "Global Public Health," 71.

2. Hamel, "Catholic Identity"; Hochman and Markham, "Love and Logic"; Panicola and Barina, "Catholic Health Care"; Mitchell and Lysaught, "Equally Strange Fruit"; Panicola, "Does Hospital and Health System Consolidation Serve."

3. Kahn and Mastroianni, "Implications of Public Health"; Childress et al., "Public Health Ethics."

4. In general, bioethics' dependence on medical institutions is a weakness for the field. Initially, bioethics was a field that drew heavily on religious ethicists and philosophers with institutional homes in their own academic departments, along with doctors, lawyers, and scientists, all with their own professional homes. As academic departments ceased hiring in bioethics, though, the field relocated to centers in hospitals, dependent on soft money grants and the goodwill of administrators. This dependence encourages bioethicists to pursue questions and answers that will ensure institutional success. For a discussion of the problems in bioethics due to its institutional structures, see Elliott, "Why Clinical Ethicists Are Not Activists." For the dangers of such grant-based incentives in research more broadly, see P. Scherz, *Science and Christian Ethics*.

5. For an institutional history of U.S. medicine, see Starr, *Social Transformation*.

6. See Starr, *Social Transformation*, and literary descriptions of the problems of medicine, such as Lewis, *Arrowsmith*.

7. For a description of these institutional changes, see Hadler, *By the Bedside*.

8. Ironically, David Rothman cites the influence of a renewed focus on the common good of the nation inspired by the experience of the wars of the twentieth century for the shift toward the utilitarian use of patients. Just as soldiers suffered on the battlefield for the common good, it was thought that patients could also serve the common good as draftees into research projects. Here again we see a population focus. See Rothman, *Strangers at the Bedside*, 48–50. For a recent discussion of criticisms of the common good in research ethics, see London, *For the Common Good*, 27–86.

9. The history of bioethics recounted here follows standard versions found in sources like Rothman, *Strangers at the Bedside*; Evans, *Playing God?*; Jonsen, *Birth of Bioethics*.

10. E.g., Ramsey, *Patient as Person*; Illich, *Limits to Medicine*.

11. E.g., Daniels, *Just Health Care*; Callahan, *Setting Limits*.

12. For a description of the treatment of the body as mechanism in the ICU, see Bishop, *Anticipatory Corpse*.

13. This dynamic is well described by Gawande, "Whose Body Is It, Anyway?"; Gawande, *Being Mortal*.

14. Dworkin, *Medical Catastrophe*, 55–76.

15. Rozier, "When Populations Become the Patient," 6; Rozier, "Religion and Public Health," 1053; Panicola, "Does Hospital and Health System Consolidation Serve."

16. Leder, *Absent Body*; McKenny, *To Relieve the Human Condition*.

17. Cassell, *Nature of Suffering*, 103–4.

18. Marmot, "Social Determinants."

19. After a long period of quiescence, these questions again became pressing in the midst of the pandemic, as hospitals sought policies to ethically distribute ventilators and other medications, and governments sought the most ethical way to distribute newly developed vaccines. See, for example, Emanuel et al., "Fair Allocation"; *Public Discourse* editors, "Moral Guidance."

20. Russell, "Prevention vs. Cure."

21. Rose, *Strategy of Preventive Medicine*, 2–4.

22. Charon, *Narrative Medicine*.

CHAPTER SIX   The Limitless Demand for Health

1. World Health Organization, "Constitution."

2. E.g., Keane, *Catholicism and Health-Care Justice*, 10–11.

3. Ewald, *État Providence*, 424ff. See also Beck, *Risk Society*.

4. Greene, *Prescribing by Numbers*, 151–220.

5. For an argument in favor of exceeding species-level norms for decreased cholesterol, see Austriaco, "Healthier Than Healthy."

6. Aristotle, *Politics* 1.9. For a similar analysis in terms of length of life, see P. Scherz, "Living Indefinitely and Living Fully." For a discussion of greed and risk with a slightly different emphasis, see P. Scherz, *Tomorrow's Troubles*, 64–70.

7. Aristotle, *Politics* 1.9, trans. Lord.

8. Greene, *Prescribing by Numbers*; Dumit, *Drugs for Life*; Kaufman, *Ordinary Medicine*.

9. Lundh et al., "Industry Sponsorship."

10. Hou et al., "Precision Medicine."

11. MacIntyre, *After Virtue*.

12. Thus the common good is reduced to basic or generic interests. London, *For the Common Good*, 131–40.

13. In the late 1970s, Michel Foucault used his lecture series at the College de France to describe the rise of what he called biopower as a mode of power that now predominates over older forms of sovereign power, even if it does not replace

them. Biopower seeks to enhance the life of citizens for state ends. Whereas sovereign power claims the right to "*take* life or *let* live," biopower makes live and lets die, the state can "*foster* life or *disallow* it" (Foucault, *History of Sexuality*, 1:138). Biopolitics, the most important aspect of biopower for this project, aims at the management of populations. See Foucault, *Society Must Be Defended*; Foucault, *Security, Territory, Population*; Foucault, *Birth of Biopolitics*; Foucault, *History of Sexuality*, vol. 1. For discussion and analysis of these texts, see P. Scherz, *Science and Christian Ethics*, 98–112.

14. Gould, *Mismeasure of Man*; Kevles, *In the Name of Eugenics*.

15. Fisher and Fisk, *How to Live*, ix.

16. Fisher and Fisk, *How to Live*, x. This conceptualization of health and social welfare reached its apogee under the Nazi racial hygiene program that aimed at maximizing the health of a population mobilized for total war. For history, see Proctor, *Racial Hygiene*. For the importance of the idea of race war in the development of biopolitics, see Foucault, *Society Must Be Defended*.

17. In a quote frequently attributed (although mistakenly) to Paul Krugman, "The US government . . . is best thought of as a giant insurance company with an army." See Krugman, "Insurance Company." The military and the insurance function are historically interrelated roles. For a discussion of the insurance role of government, see P. Scherz, *Tomorrow's Troubles*, 93–116, 200.

18. For the political problems of interventions creating risk, see the literature on the risk society, including Beck, *Risk Society*; Luhmann, *Risk*; Beck, *World at Risk*.

19. For a deeper discussion, see P. Scherz, "No Acceptable Losses."

20. For a description of the problems of this kind of science, see Weinberg, "Science and Trans-science"; P. Scherz, *Science and Christian Ethics*, 151–73.

21. That is not to say that a researcher could not design complex cluster-randomized controlled trials to test many of these questions, but they are large-scale and expensive. For example, the Bangladesh Study of the efficacy of masking against Covid-19 involved 342,183 adults from nearly six hundred villages. See Abaluck et al., "Impact of Community Masking."

22. Proctor and Schiebinger, *Agnotology*; Oreskes and Conway, *Merchants of Doubt*.

23. A good discussion of the conceptual difficulties of pricing subjective factors can be found in Shrader-Frechette, *Science Policy*. An explanation and defense of different methods of pricing life-years is Sunstein, *Laws of Fear*. For a descriptions of the problems with QALYs and DALYs, see Anand and Hanson, "Disability-Adjusted Life Years"; Brock, "Ethical Issues."

24. Welch, Schwartz, and Woloshin, *Overdiagnosed*, 74–77; O'Callaghan, "Mammogram Recommendations."

25. Ewald, *État Providence*, 424.

26. This is the fundamental insight of Agamben's integration of Carl Schmitt's notions of sovereignty into the Foucaultian analysis of biopolitics in Agamben, *Homo Sacer*. Ultimately the ground for these decisions on acceptable risk becomes sovereign power, as clearly shown in the pandemic. It was the executive power, operating outside legislative authority, that decided the limits to public health action, as articulated in Agamben, *Where Are We Now?* Courts did eventually limit executive authority, but for a long time countries operated in the state of exception described in Schmitt, *Political Theology*; Agamben, *State of Exception*. See also Kheriaty, *New Abnormal*.

In this case, as in many other aspects of our contemporary world, the sovereign is not some single political figure. Instead, sovereignty lies within the technocracy of public health administration. Agamben obliquely discusses the distinction between law and administration in Agamben, "Kingdom and the Glory."

CHAPTER SEVEN   Managing Populations

1. Hudson and Pollitz, "Undermining Genetic Privacy?"

2. For the complex ways to calculate the optimal valuation of life years, see Sunstein, *Laws of Fear*.

3. E.g., Daniels, *Just Health Care*; Callahan, *Setting Limits*; Camosy, *Too Expensive to Treat?*; Lustig, "Reform and Rationing."

4. For an analysis of the CMS's approval process and the way it shapes healthcare cost and patient experience, see Kaufman, *Ordinary Medicine*.

5. Rose, *Strategy of Preventive Medicine*, 2–4; Russell, "Prevention vs. Cure."

6. This is not to say that risk reduction is the sole driver of costs. It is not. In most discussions, prevention serves as a response to the rising costs of salaries, surgeries, price gouging, the overuse of expensive technologies, etc.

7. Hadler, *Worried Sick*.

8. For overviews of VBC, see Berwick, Nolan, and Whittington, "Triple Aim"; Berkovich and Sitipati, *Applied Population Health*; Mjåset et al., "Value-Based Health Care." For criticism of other aspects of VBC, see P. Scherz, "Data Ethics."

9. Berwick, "Making Good."

10. Kahneman, *Thinking, Fast and Slow*; Gigerenzer, *Rationality for Mortals*.

11. Mol, *Logic of Care*.

12. Pellegrino and Thomasma, *Philosophical Basis*; Cassell, *Nature of Suffering*; Mol, *Logic of Care*.

13. Juengst et al., "From 'Personalized' to 'Precision' Medicine."

14. Berwick, "Making Good."

15. Swensen et al., "Cottage Industry," e12(3). This discussion of the problem of using process measures and their impingement on clinical judgment draws on the analysis found in Mutter, "New Stranger." For discussion of another risk reduction program, one focusing on suicide prevention, on the healing relationship, see Kinghorn, "Protecting Life."

16. Sarosi, "Tyranny of Guidelines."

17. Mutter, "New Stranger."

18. Babic et al., "Beware Explanations."

19. W. Price, Gerke, and Cohen, "Potential Liability."

20. Carr, *Glass Cage*; Perrow, *Normal Accidents*; Mouloua and Parasuraman, *Automation and Human Performance*.

21. Zigon, "Can Machines Be Ethical?"; P. Scherz, *Tomorrow's Troubles*, chap. 8.

22. Berwick, "Health Services Research," 661.

23. P. Scherz, "Data Ethics."

24. "Judge Blocks New York City Large-Soda Ban." Framing opposition to this rule in terms of consumer autonomy ignores efforts of soda companies to manipulate behavior through marketing. It also ignores the role agricultural subsidies play in making high-fructose corn syrup, and thus soda, cheaper. See Pollan, *Omnivore's Dilemma*.

25. P. Scherz, *Tomorrow's Troubles*, 117–61.

26. See the discussion of the increasing prominence of biosecurity as a political paradigm in Agamben, *Where Are We Now?*; Kheriaty, *New Abnormal*.

CHAPTER EIGHT   The Obligation of Health

1. My aim in this section is not to prove this obligation, which I am taking as a premise, but just to suggest that it is broadly recognized by many in our society, even those who may not explicitly describe it as a normative obligation.

2. Thaler and Sunstein, *Nudge*.

3. Stanley Hauerwas describes the confusion of medical students committed to principles of autonomy when asked what justified their reviving a suicide victim in the emergency room in Hauerwas, *Suffering Presence*, 100–101.

4. E.g., Grisez, "First Principle"; Finnis, "Practical Reasoning"; Foot, *Natural Goodness*.

5. The fundamental modern source for this casuistical tradition with regard to duties of preserving health is this historical analysis found in Cronin, *Ordinary and Extraordinary Means*. See also G. Kelly, "Duty of Using Artificial Means"; G. Kelly, "Duty to Preserve Life."

6. Cronin, *Ordinary and Extraordinary Means*, 4–46.

7. John Paul II, *Evangelium Vitae*, 41.
8. Crislip, *From Monastery to Hospital*; Ferngren, *Medicine and Health Care*.
9. Cronin, *Ordinary and Extraordinary Means*, 48–108.
10. Cronin, *Ordinary and Extraordinary Means*, 130–33.
11. Cronin, *Ordinary and Extraordinary Means*, 41–44, 139–46.
12. The main issue debated in recent times with regard to this obligation of ordinary care is the provision of artificial nutrition and hydration (ANH), especially for patients in a persistent vegetative state (PVS). This debate is the exception that proves the rule. The controversy is primarily about making decisions for a patient who cannot herself decide because of PVS, coma, Alzheimer's, or another condition, who therefore cannot make her own prudential judgment. It is also a debate as to what ANH is: whether it is more akin to normal feeding or to a ventilator. Finally, even when the Vatican ruled that ANH is an ordinary, proportionate means of preserving life, it still left open the possibility that ANH could become burdensome in particular cases. For these discussions, see articles in Hamel and Walter, *Artificial Nutrition and Hydration*.

Giorgio Agamben uses cases of people in a PVS to demonstrate the separation of bare life from social existence, arguing that it traps the person in an asocial boundary situation (Agamben, *Homo Sacer*; Agamben, *Where Are We Now?*). He may have a point in terms of brain death and some scholarly discussions of PVS, but his reading of the Catholic tradition is inaccurate. According to many Catholic bioethicists, it is through the provision of food and water, even artificially, that caregivers maintain social bonds with the patient and demonstrate the patient's continued role in the community as wife, husband, son, daughter, father, or mother (e.g., Grisez, "Should Nutrition and Hydration Be Provided"). In contrast to Agamben's reading, ANH maintains solidarity. Take the example of Mr. Sato in Kaufman, *And a Time to Die*. Through his continued care of his wife, Sylvia, who is in a long-term coma, he affected how the nursing staff viewed her: "Mr. Sato's unwavering hope and sense of duty define Mrs. Sato as a valuable person with a potential future, a social being connected by love and personal history to him and to family. . . . Though she lies curled on her side in a hospital bed, unresponsive . . . Mrs. Sato is, to her husband and perhaps to the nurses, a whole person" (299). Bodily care is a part of our social obligations and is invested with meaning and dignity.

13. Cronin, *Ordinary and Extraordinary Means*, 60.
14. Congregation for the Doctrine of the Faith, "Note on the Morality."
15. Barilan, *Jewish Bioethics*, 46–49.
16. Barilan, *Jewish Bioethics*, 46.
17. Austriaco, *Biomedicine and Beatitude*, 221. He embraces this argument to avoid possible moral problems with risk-reducing prophylactic surgeries that

also sterilize the patient. For criticism of his position, see Barina, "Prophylactic Salpingectomy."

18. Eberl, "Thomistic Appraisal," 301.
19. Austriaco, "Healthier Than Healthy," 46.
20. Austriaco, "Healthier Than Healthy," 47.
21. Austriaco, "Healthier Than Healthy," 46.
22. Austriaco, "Healthier Than Healthy," 48.
23. Cataldo, "Why the CDF 'Note'"; Eberl and Winright, "Catholics Have No Grounds"; Lysaught, "Catholics Seeking 'Religious' Exemptions"; Eberl, "Is There a Moral Obligation?"
24. I made these arguments in the winter and spring of 2021, when most of the population had not been infected with Covid and on the basis of the clinical trial results, which showed relatively mild side effects. Primarily, I sought to ease worries of the dangers of cooperation with evil due to the use of cell lines derived from abortion in vaccine development. See Institute for Human Ecology, "COVID Vaccine"; P. Scherz, "Are Immortalized Cell Lines Artifacts?"

These arguments are still valid, although the situation has changed now that most of the population has been either vaccinated or infected and rare side effects have been identified among specific subpopulations for particular vaccines (e.g., VITT in young women or myocarditis in young men). Thus the guidelines of many European nations, like the U.K. and Scandinavian nations, which recommend booster vaccinations only for high-risk groups, like older adults, seem prudent at this stage of the disease (e.g., National Health Service, "Getting a COVID-19 Vaccine"; Public Health Agency of Sweden, "COVID-19 Recommendations"). Such recommendations need to be responsive to new evidence, changing situations, and up-to-date risk analysis.

25. For these arguments, see P. Scherz, "Risk, Health"; C. Kelly, "On Pediatric Vaccines."
26. For opposition to the idea of an obligation for Covid vaccination based on different premises from my own, see Camosy, "Clearing Up"; Janet Smith, "Fake Theology"; R. Anderson et al., "Open Letter"; Kheriaty, *New Abnormal*.
27. Eberl's translations from Eberl and Winright, "Catholics Have No Grounds"; Eberl, "Is There a Moral Obligation."
28. This is the reason that ANH is considered obligatory in general for those who have lost the ability to eat in the normal way. The broader context of Aquinas's commentary suggests that this obligation refers to the need to work to obtain food.
29. For example, the risk for a child or a twenty-something is orders of magnitude lower than for an older adult, which would seem to affect this obligation. See Centers for Disease Control, "Risk for COVID-19 Infection." These authors also ignore the questions of those previously infected, and so on.

30. See the foundational discussions on the problem of the binding force of secular obligation in Anscombe, "Modern Moral Philosophy." She, and others following her, turn to virtue to solve these problems of the ground of moral obligation, but that turn is unlikely to work in this case. As my argument thus far suggests, it is far from clear that this kind of micromanagement of health is virtuous.

31. For discussion of contemporary secular moral demands surrounding health, see Lupton, *Imperative of Health*; Metzl and Kirkland, *Against Health*. For Foucault's concept of governmentality, which inspired these analyses, see Foucault et al., *Foucault Effect*; Dean, *Governmentality*; O'Malley, "Governmentality and Risk"; Foucault, *Security, Territory, Population*; Foucault, *Birth of Biopolitics*.

32. This is part of the broader project of forming a responsible citizenry, as critiqued in Mounk, *Age of Responsibility*. For the background to the drive by contemporary power to encourage individuals to internalize others' ends, see Dean, *Governmentality*; Foucault et al., *Foucault Effect*; Gane, "Foucault on Governmentality"; O'Malley, "Governmentality and Risk"; Foucault, *Security, Territory, Population*; Foucault, *Birth of Biopolitics*.

33. Metzl and Kirkland, *Against Health*.

34. Plato, *Laws* 406c–407.

35. Ehrenreich, *Natural Causes*, 2.

CHAPTER NINE   Exclusion and Elimination

1. Rose, *Strategy of Preventive Medicine*, 95–106.

2. Rose, *Strategy of Preventive Medicine*, 29–52.

3. In its possible focus on the marginalized, it embodies the preferential option for the poor, a principle of Catholic social teaching derived from liberation theology. For its roots in Catholic social teaching, see Paul VI, *Octogesima Adveniens*. The preferential option for the poor has also been embraced by global health activists like Farmer, *Pathologies of Power*. The reasons to support a preferential option for the poor include the fact that disease itself preferentially strikes the poor, as the social determinants of health demonstrate. Further, policies can frequently have disproportionate impact by focusing on the poor. Finally, in a theological vein, Christians should emulate God, who hears the cry of the poor.

4. Behforouz et al., "Directly Observed Therapy"; Shin et al., "Community-Based Treatment."

5. For these programs, see Gawande, "Hot Spotters"; Thomas-Henkel, Hamblin, and Hendricks, "Supporting a Culture of Health."

6. P. Scherz, "Data Ethics."

7. Pope Francis has described this broader tendency as an aspect of the throwaway culture, in which the vulnerable are excluded. For an examination of this concept in relation to bioethics, see Camosy, *Resisting Throwaway Culture*.

8. Giorgio Agamben emphasizes that exclusion is a basic feature of biopolitical governance. The most important figure in his thought is *homo sacer*, the sacred man of Roman law who could be killed but not sacrificed. The declaration of "*Sacer esto*" cursed a person who committed a sacrilegious act. That person became accursed and excluded from society, put under the ban. See Agamben, *Homo Sacer*.

The figure of the excluded *homo sacer* was Agamben's addition to Foucault's definition of biopolitics as the power of making live and letting die. People who are rejected from the programs of the state are left to die in biopolitics. What Agamben helpfully points to is the ambiguity of their position: such people are related to the population (in my example as being at the highest risk) but are excluded from governmental mechanisms because of their failure to respond to risk reduction. Yet in their existence as the highest risk that is excluded, they demonstrate the system's basic mechanism of power, which consists in the indefinite reduction of risk. These patients are the most important target of state power but also end up excluded by it. My analysis adds to Agamben's by highlighting the role statistical quantification of population risk plays in these political phenomena.

9. Life insurance is one of the realms in which genetic information can still be used against a person under U.S. law. The Genetic Information Nondiscrimination Act (GINA) does not cover life insurance. See National Human Genome Research Institute, "Genetic Discrimination."

10. Bouk, *How Our Days Became Numbered*; Ewald, *État Providence*. See also P. Scherz, *Tomorrow's Troubles*, 93–116.

11. There is another, positive eugenic strategy not based in risk and fear that can serve as a helpful comparison to the risk reduction paradigm. In this vision, genetics and eugenics programs would identify exceptional members of the population and encourage their fertility. This vision lay behind Galton's book *Hereditary Genius*, the "Fitter Families" competitions of the eugenics era, and the "Repository for Germinal Choice," a sperm bank that allowed only sperm donors who were geniuses. Here policymakers focused on expanding the ranks of those at low risk rather than eliminating those at high risk. It is also worth noting the risk paradigm's difference from 1960s fears about the growing load of genetic mutations. Geneticists generally confronted this danger by encouraging genetic engineering rather than eugenic selection. See Ramsey, *Fabricated Man*; Kaye, *Social Meaning*.

12. Savulescu, "Procreative Beneficence"; Agar, *Liberal Eugenics*.

13. McKeown, *Modern Rise of Population*.

14. McKeown, *Modern Rise of Population*, 168.

15. As the example of an obstinate will, take Dostoevsky's Underground Man, who will shake his fist at the Crystal Palace of progress. See Dostoevsky, *Notes from Underground*, 18.

16. One can see a similar temporal difference in the mechanisms of sovereignty and biopolitical power as described by Foucault. Sovereign power kills or lets live. It kills generally in response to past or present action. For sovereign power, death and life are in the present. Biopolitics is oriented toward the future. It makes live and lets die. It organizes the continuation of life through programs of risk reduction oriented toward future danger. Or it excludes high-risk or nonresponsive individuals from its programs, allowing them to drift toward a future death.

CHAPTER TEN   Caring for the Statistical Other

1. Ferngren, *Medicine and Health Care*, 115–23.
2. Cyprian, *Mortality* 14, trans. Deferrari.
3. Cyprian, *Mortality* 14, trans. Deferrari.
4. Francis, "Moment of Prayer." Ultimately, of course, the good aimed at is eternal life. It is this final end that allows Christians to accept temporal disaster and risk to health.
5. Cyprian, *Mortality* 16, trans. Deferrari.
6. P. Scherz, "Grief, Death, and Longing."
7. Pontius the Deacon, "Life and Passion of Cyprian," chap. 9, trans. Wallis.
8. Cyprian, *Mortality* 16, trans. Deferrari.
9. Ferngren, *Medicine and Health Care*.
10. Pope Francis called on Catholics to emulate this same freedom from fear in the homily that accompanied his special *Urbi et Orbi* blessing early in the pandemic. For Francis as well, the pandemic has served to reveal our selfishness. "Greedy for profit, we let ourselves get caught up in things, and lured away by haste." The answer is to turn to others, to "put into practice that solidarity and hope capable of giving strength, support and meaning to these hours when everything seems to be floundering." Such concrete acts of care are part of building a culture of encounter that Francis has frequently called for, a culture of interpersonal engagement and care. He notes those who engaged others in the pandemic: doctors, nurses, other medical staff, cleaners, supermarket employees, and so forth. See Francis, "Moment of Prayer."
11. Note that am I not claiming that such a response can be found only in Christian texts; these texts themselves draw on Stoic and Jewish precedents, so clearly these tenets are found in other philosophical and religious groups.

12. Dickenson, *Me Medicine*. Dickenson fears that precision medicine might reinforce the advantages of the wealthy by giving them the ability to manage their own health. She suggests using precision medicine to benefit the broader community. See also Prainsack and Buyx, *Solidarity in Biomedicine*; Prainsack, *Personalized Medicine*.

13. For example, the English translation of Francois Ewald's philosophical history of the welfare state is entitled *The Birth of Solidarity*. See Ewald, *Birth of Solidarity*; Ewald, *État Providence*. Yet even with regard to social insurance, claims of a growth in solidarity through socialization are questionable. Daniel Defert describes how the friendly societies that provided insurance as well as other forms of social support to their small groups of members opposed the attempts by insurance companies and the state to usurp their insurance functions. See Defert, "'Popular Life'"; P. Scherz, *Tomorrow's Troubles*, chaps. 6, 11. The true solidarity and common action of these independent groups was lost to centralized management.

Richard Titmuss describes the solidarity, reciprocity, and altruism shaped by social services, like the U.K.'s National Health Service, in Titmuss, *Gift Relationship*. Yet his example of voluntary blood donation demonstrated a broad reciprocity toward individual others. These donations were concrete gifts by the self or from others rather than the manipulation of abstract population figures, so they seem like a different sort of relationship from the population health described here. Moreover, the feelings of solidarity tied to blood donation drew on a richer fund of nationalistic feeling formed through the experience of World War II, as described in Titmuss's own interview data and in Paul Rabinow's description of blood donation in France. See Titmuss, *Gift Relationship*, 230–32; Rabinow, *French DNA*.

14. Prainsack and Buyx describe a number of scholarly definitions of solidarity in Prainsack and Buyx, *Solidarity in Biomedicine*. They settle on a threefold typology of solidarity: interpersonal solidarity, group solidarity, and solidarity in law. While I find their analysis helpful, I will discuss solidarity normatively in terms of the interpersonal level as a virtue. Their focus on practices that enhance solidarity is extremely useful. See also the multiple frameworks of solidarity described in Stjernø, *Solidarity in Europe*.

15. John Paul II, *Sollicitudo Rei Socialis*.

16. Aristotle, *Nicomachean Ethics* 8.9.

17. My discussion in this paragraph relies heavily on the interpretation of Hittinger, "Coherence." To fully embrace this concept, one needs to also accept the idea that ordered social groupings, what are called societies, can establish their own form of moral personhood. They have an independent status, end, and value beyond what is granted by the state and beyond merely individual volition.

18. Classic sources for this debate include Schelling, "Life You Save"; Fried, "Value of Life"; Jonsen, "Bentham in a Box." For an excellent overview of

contemporary arguments, see Cohen, Daniels, and Eyal, *Identified versus Statistical Lives*.

19. Brock, "Identified versus Statistical Lives," 49.
20. Fried, "Value of Life," 1436–37; Slote, "Why Not Empathy?"
21. Jonsen, "Bentham in a Box."
22. Pellegrino and Thomasma make a similar argument that certain forms of rationing medical care are acceptable, but it is imperative that the doctor not be the one to make rationing decisions. That kind of prioritization of the social good over the patient would undermine the healing relationship. See Pellegrino and Thomasma, *For the Patient's Good*, 177–80.
23. Verweij, "How (Not) to Argue."
24. For Ferdinand Tonnies, the difference between the organic solidaristic relationship that he sees in *Gemeinschaft* and the individualistic outlook found in the association-form of *Gesellschaft* arises because of abstraction. Commercial society abstracts from concrete relationship by basing all interactions on money. Similarly, population statistics engage the same process of abstraction, not through money but through statistics. See Tonnies, *Community and Civil Society*.
25. Hence the military's emphasis on leaving no man behind.
26. This discussion draws on Farmer, "Chronic Infectious Disease." See also Kidder, *Mountains beyond Mountains*.
27. E.g., Marseille, Hofmann, and Kahn, "HIV Prevention before HAART."
28. Epstein, *Invisible Cure*.
29. Agamben, *Homo Sacer*; Arendt, *Human Condition*. These authors distinguish *bios* from *zoe*. *Bios* is our social form of life, such as being a philosopher or political actor. Ancient authors were largely concerned with *bios*. *Zoe* refers to our animal existence, our basic needs. In Aristotle, *zoe* was solely a matter for the home. Over time, the emphasis changes, driven by the late antique embrace of the term *zoe* and by the Christian exaltation of individual life directed toward eternal life. Following a long process of change, modern states now embrace only the maintenance of biological existence. For these later shifts, see Agamben, "Use of Bodies," 1221–27.
30. Partners in Health has been criticized for doing this in some of its messaging by Butt, "Suffering Stranger." See the more general criticism of the spectacle entailed in the media's depiction of humanitarianism in Boltanski, *Distant Suffering*. My point is that we need to see others in their richer social context, in terms of the fullness of life, not merely as either statistical data points or abstract idealizations of suffering.
31. For this ethics of encounter, especially as it is elaborated by Pope Francis, see Pope, "Integral Human Development"; Mescher, *Ethics of Encounter*; P. Scherz, "Data Ethics."

CHAPTER ELEVEN   Prevention and the Social Determinants of Health

1. Rose, *Strategy of Preventive Medicine*, 94–95. My analysis in general in this chapter is deeply influenced by Rose's work.
2. Rose, *Strategy of Preventive Medicine*, 94.
3. See also Potter, *Bioethics*.
4. Oreskes and Conway, *Merchants of Doubt*; Proctor and Schiebinger, *Agnotology*; Proctor, *Golden Holocaust*; P. Scherz, *Science and Christian Ethics*, 151–73. Corporate pressure with regard to environmental dangers is well established, but there can be just as much ideological pressure against investigating long-term effects of transgender surgeries, IVF, or marijuana.
5. Rose, *Strategy of Preventive Medicine*, 107–29; McKeown, *Modern Rise of Population*; Marmot, "Social Determinants"; Marmot, *Health Gap*.
6. Bosma et al., "Two Alternative Job Stress Models"; Ferrie et al., "Uncertain Future"; Head et al., "Influence of Change"; László et al., "Job Insecurity and Health"; Kivimäki et al., "Individual and Combined Effects"; Taouk et al., "All-Cause Mortality."
7. For discussions of the dire conditions of contemporary work, see Graeber, *Bullshit Jobs*; Cloutier, "Worker's Paradise."
8. Davis, "Devalued Status," 31–33.
9. Badal et al., "Prediction of Loneliness."
10. The disempowering of the individual citizen is one of the foundations of Ivan Illich's critique of what he calls the disabling professions. See Illich, *Deschooling Society*; Illich, Zola, and McKnight, *Disabling Professions*; Illich, *Limits to Medicine*. He also thinks these professions create the experience of new needs among otherwise stable populations by generating a hope that is impossible to fulfill. This latter aspect of his critique relates to my analysis of the expansive nature of risk reduction that ultimately seems to promise the eradication of risk, and thus of death itself.
11. Pollan, *Omnivore's Dilemma*.
12. Scott, *Seeing Like a State*.
13. Rozier, "Collective Action."
14. With regard to the influence of healthcare corporations on NGOs in population health, see L. Taylor, "How Do We Fund Flourishing?" For similar criticisms to the one found here on the role of population health in social problems, see Lantz, "Medicalization of Population Health"; Lantz, "'Super-utilizer' Interventions."
15. The most insightful scholars in public health policy recognize this. Rozier, for example, argues that Catholic health systems must let other Catholic apostolates take a leading role in addressing social issues. See Rozier, "Collective Action."

CHAPTER TWELVE   Regimen

1. For a recent secular account of habits, see Clear, *Atomic Habits*. For a theological and virtue-based approach, see E. Sullivan, *Habits and Holiness*; Mattison, *Growing in Virtue*.

2. Foucault, *Use of Pleasure*, 99–108; Foucault, *Care of the Self*, 99–104.

3. For overviews of ancient medicine, see Craik, *"Hippocratic" Corpus*; Nutton, *Ancient Medicine*; Temkin, *Galenism*. Admittedly, the Hippocratic Corpus was much less focused on the humors than Galen. Only a few of this diverse set of treatises used humoral theory. Still, the vision of Hippocratic medicine that later developed, encouraged by Galen, was humoral.

4. Scrinis, "On the Ideology."

5. Plato, *Laws*.

6. Pollan, *Omnivore's Dilemma*.

7. Bourdieu, *Distinction*.

8. Bourdieu, *Distinction*, 194.

9. Bourdieu, *Distinction*, 197.

10. Bourdieu, *Distinction*, 196.

11. Wolf, "Futurist Ray Kurzweil."

12. For his theory of technological immortality, see Kurzweil, *Singularity Is Near*.

13. P. Scherz, "Grief, Death, and Longing"; P. Scherz, "Living Indefinitely."

14. Foucault, *Courage of Truth*.

15. Plato, *Republic* 403c–407, trans. Hutchinson, 1040–44. For discussion, see McKenny, *To Relieve the Human Condition*, 1.

16. Miller, *Arete*, 174–77.

17. Edelstein, "Dietetics of Antiquity."

18. Schull, "Data-Based Self."

19. Foucault, *Hermeneutics of the Subject*; Foucault, *Care of the Self*.

20. Foucault, *Use of Pleasure*, 103.

21. For a good discussion of Clement in terms of practices and ethics, see Brown, *Body and Society*, 122–39.

22. Clement of Alexandria, *Christ the Educator*, trans. Wood, 88.

23. Clement of Alexandria, *Christ the Educator*, trans. Wood, 94–97.

24. Clement of Alexandria, *Christ the Educator*, trans. Wood, 159–64.

25. Clement of Alexandria, *Christ the Educator*, trans. Wood, 237–38.

26. See, for example, the discussion in Macrobius, *Commentary on the Dream of Scipio*.

27. Aquinas, *Summa Theologica* I-II.63a4, trans. Dominicans.

28. Aquinas, *Summa Theologica* I-II.61a5, trans. Dominicans.

29. Giorgio Agamben, building on Foucault's work on the stylization of life through the care of the self, turns to the concept of a form-of-life as a way to reject the separation of *bios* from *zoe* that is at the heart of biopolitics in Agamben, "Highest Poverty"; Agamben, "Use of Bodies." He develops it from monastic practice, ultimately from Franciscan ideals. The whole of one's life, including the regimen that cares for basic functions, is to aim at a purpose, even if that purpose is only the demonstration of an ideal. Health is a subordinate goal, and bare life is not considered.

30. E.g., Coblentz, "Catholic Fasting Literature."

31. The overaestheticism of asceticism is one of the most frequently voiced critiques of the late Foucault's aesthetics of existence, which draws on these ancient sources. See Hadot, *Philosophy*, 206–12; Szakolczai, *Max Weber*, 59. Foucault's late works opened into alternative directions, either philosophy as a form of life oriented toward truth or a seemingly California-inspired obsession with lifestyle for its own sake. For a defense of Foucault's interpretation of ancient ascetic practice as necessitating an orientation toward truth, see P. Scherz, *Science and Christian Ethics*, 174–89.

32. Cassian, *Conferences*, trans. Ramsey, 99–104; Benedict, *Rule of Saint Benedict*, chaps. 39–40.

33. Cassian, *Conferences*, trans. Ramsey, 603–4, 731–37.

34. Crislip, *From Monastery to Hospital*.

35. Rebillard, *In hora mortis*, 185–96.

36. Indeed, caloric restriction seems to be one of the surest ways to increase longevity.

CHAPTER THIRTEEN   Genomics in the Identification and Treatment of Disease

1. For discussion, see Grob, *Testing Baby*, 39–79.

2. 100,000 Genomes Project Pilot Investigators, "100,000 Genomes Pilot."

3. 100,000 Genomes Project Pilot Investigators, "100,000 Genomes Pilot," 1875.

4. "Gene Therapies Should Be for All"; Walker, "FDA Approves"; McPhillips, "FDA Approves."

5. Feuerstein, "Bluebird's Withdrawal of Therapy."

6. See, for example, Eva Kittay's discussion of the benefits of finding other parents of children with the same condition as her daughter in Kittay, "We Have Seen the Mutants," S51–52. This is one example of the new social formations

arising from genetic or medically based solidarity, as described in Rabinow, "Artificiality and Enlightenment."

7. As earlier chapters noted, though, such advocacy efforts can also lead to problems when they become overly focused on prevention.

8. Breastcancer.org, "Breast Cancer Facts."

9. Sawyers, "Herceptin."

10. Nogrady, "How Cancer Genomics Is Transforming." See broader discussion of AI and genomics in Topol, *Deep Medicine*.

11. Schwarze et al., "Complete Costs."

12. For discussion of clinical trials surrounding precision medicine and their failures, see Prasad, *Malignant*.

13. Haslam et al., "Umbrella Review."

14. Hey et al., "Evidence Landscape."

15. For a review of these problems in current scientific research, see P. Scherz, *Science and Christian Ethics*.

16. For a discussion of how large a margin of benefit needs to be to justify a preventive intervention, see Hadler, *Last Well Person*.

17. Gibson, "On the Utilization."

18. James et al., "Limits of Personalization."

19. Muller, *Tyranny of Metrics*.

20. Babic et al., "Beware Explanations."

21. National Cancer Insitute, "Cancer Moonshot[SM]."

22. R. Sullivan et al., "Global Cancer Surgery."

23. Zubizarreta et al., "Need for Radiotherapy."

24. Gyawali, Sullivan, and Booth, "Cancer Groundshot."

CHAPTER FOURTEEN Institutions for Slow Medicine

1. This description relies on C. Scherz, *Having People*; C. Scherz, "Let Us Make God Our Banker"; C. Scherz, "Enduring the Awkward Embrace." Mercy House is a pseudonym. Although I was present for most of my wife's fieldwork at Mercy House, and I continue to be friends with many of the sisters, I use published data rather than personal memories in order to protect the site's anonymity.

2. See similar challenges to Ghanaian prayer camps for the mentally ill described in Goldstone, "Prayer's Chance." In contrast to those camps, Mercy House provided good, modern medical care.

3. Crislip, *From Monastery to Hospital*; Ferngren, *Medicine and Health Care*.

4. Sweet, *God's Hotel*.

5. Stegenga, *Medical Nihilism*.

6. For a deeper exploration of logics of care and their connection to the provision of time for discussing the details of procedures and therapies with patients, see Mol, *Logic of Care*.

7. For a description of this revolving-door pathway, see Kaufman, *And a Time to Die*, 131–46.

8. Such spaces are unintelligible even to critics of modern bureaucratic institutions like Ivan Illich and Charles Taylor. Both scholars argue that the kinds of institutions I criticize in the rest of the book initially stem from a corruption of Christianity. In their view, the early church made a mistake when it attempted to institutionalize charity through hospitals and organized diocesan poor relief (Cayley and Taylor, *Rivers North*; C. Taylor, *Secular Age*, 737–42). These new social forms undermined the aspect of free encounter so necessary for the charity that one sees in the parable of the Good Samaritan. Instead, charitable care becomes technical and bureaucratic.

While recognizing the potential failings of such institutions, I disagree with their diagnosis. I have seen and read too many examples of encounter and accompaniment occurring at institutions like Mercy House. Instead, I would argue that the problem arises when institutions of care start to run on a logic of quantitative optimization and efficiency. Pre- or early modern institutions rarely did so, and they provided space for those who needed long-term care that was otherwise difficult to provide by any one member of the community.

9. Braswell, *Crisis of US Hospice Care*.

10. Sachs, *End of Poverty*; Singer, *Life You Can Save*. Medical anthropologists and critics of development have chronicled the increasing influence of technological solutionism. Funders provide pharmaceuticals or vaccines for a specific disease like HIV or malaria rather than funding for a healthcare system. Any system-level investment is tied to technologies like apps. This has led to the continued deterioration of health systems across the Global South. See Benton, *HIV Exceptionalism*; Pfeiffer and Chapman, "Anthropology of Aid"; Redfield, "Fluid Technologies."

11. Mt 26:11; Mk 14:7; Jn 12:11.

12. Finkelstein et al., "Health Care Hotspotting"; Iovan et al., "Interventions to Decrease Use."

13. See, for example, Sweet, *God's Hotel*, 80–85.

14. Foucault, *History of Madness*; James Smith, *Ireland's Magdalen Laundries*.

15. Foucault, *History of Madness*, 44–77.

16. Goffman, *Asylums*; Foucault, *Discipline and Punish*.

17. C. Scherz, "Enduring the Awkward Embrace."

18. Braswell, *Crisis of US Hospice Care*.
19. Catholic healthcare systems, however, do try to provide formation in their mission to all of their staff. It is not at the same intensity as in the example of sisters, though, usually consisting of trainings.
20. Tollefson, "These Experiments."

BIBLIOGRAPHY

Abaluck, Jason, Laura H. Kwong, Ashley Styczynski, Ashraful Haque, Alamgir Kabir, Ellen Bates-Jefferys, Emily Crawford, et al. "Impact of Community Masking on COVID-19: A Cluster-Randomized Trial in Bangladesh." *Science* 375, no. 6577 (December 2, 2021): eabi9069. https://doi.org/10.1126/science.abi9069.
Agamben, Giorgio. "The Highest Poverty: Monastic Rules and Form-of-Life." In *The Omnibus Homo Sacer*, 881–1009. Stanford, CA: Stanford University Press, 2017.
———. *Homo Sacer: Sovereign Power and Bare Life*. Translated by Daniel Heller-Roazen. Stanford, CA: Stanford University Press, 1998.
———. "The Kingdom and the Glory: For a Theological Genealogy of Economy and Government." In *The Omnibus Homo Sacer*, 363–642. Stanford, CA: Stanford University Press, 2017.
———. *State of Exception*. Translated by Kevin Attell. Chicago: University of Chicago Press, 2005.
———. "The Use of Bodies." In *The Omnibus Homo Sacer*, 1011–1290. Stanford, CA: Stanford University Press, 2017.
———. *Where Are We Now? The Epidemic as Politics*. Lanham, MD: Rowman and Littlefield, 2021.
Agar, Nicholas. *Liberal Eugenics: In Defence of Human Enhancement*. Malden, MA: Wiley-Blackwell, 2004.
Alexander, Denis. *Genes, Determinism, and God*. Cambridge: Cambridge University Press, 2017.
Allen, John F. "Hypothesis, Induction and Background Knowledge: Data Do Not Speak for Themselves. Replies to Donald A. Gillies, Lawrence A. Kelly and Michael Scott." *BioEssays* 23, no. 9 (2001): 861–62. https://doi.org/10.1002/bies.1125.
All of Us. "Genomic Variants: Participant Demographics." Accessed January 24, 2023. https://databrowser.researchallofus.org/genomic-variants. Web page no longer accessible.

Anand, Sudhir, and Kara Hanson. "Disability-Adjusted Life Years: A Critical Review." In *Public Health, Ethics, and Equity*, edited by Sudhir Anand, Fabienne Peter, and Amartya Sen, 183–200. Oxford: Oxford University Press, 2004.

Anderson, Chris. "The End of Theory: The Data Deluge Makes the Scientific Method Obsolete." *WIRED* magazine, June 23, 2008. www.wired.com/2008/06/pb-theory/.

Anderson, Ryan, Aaron Kheriaty, Aaron Rothstein, Roger Severino, and Rachel Morrison. "An Open Letter to HHS Secretary Becerra on Ending the Covid-19 Public Health 'Emergency.'" *Public Discourse* (blog), March 18, 2022. www.thepublicdiscourse.com/2022/03/81209/.

Angrist, Misha. *Here Is a Human Being: At the Dawn of Personal Genomics*. New York: Harper Perennial, 2011.

Ann Arbor Science for the People Editorial Collective. *Biology as a Social Weapon*. Minneapolis, MN: Burgess, 1977.

Annas, Julia. *The Morality of Happiness*. New York: Oxford University Press, 1993.

Anscombe, G. E. M. "Modern Moral Philosophy." *Philosophy* 33, no. 124 (1958): 1–16.

Aquinas, Thomas. *Summa Theologica*. Translated by Dominicans of the English Province. New York: Benziger Bros., 1947.

Arendt, Hannah. *The Human Condition*. Chicago: University of Chicago Press, 1998.

Aristotle. *Nicomachean Ethics*. Translated by Terence Irwin. 2nd ed. Indianapolis, IN: Hackett, 1999.

———. *On the Soul*. In *A New Aristotle Reader*, edited by J. L. Ackrill, translated by D. W. Hamlyn, 161–205. Princeton, NJ: Princeton University Press, 1987.

———. *Politics*. Translated by Carnes Lord. Chicago: University of Chicago Press, 2013.

Aronowitz, Robert. *Risky Medicine: Our Quest to Cure Fear and Uncertainty*. Chicago: University of Chicago Press, 2015.

———. *Unnatural History: Breast Cancer and American Society*. New York: Cambridge University Press, 2013.

Austriaco, Nicanor Pier Giorgio. *Biomedicine and Beatitude: An Introduction to Catholic Bioethics*. Washington, DC: Catholic University of America Press, 2011.

———. "Healthier Than Healthy: The Moral Case for Therapeutic Enhancement." *National Catholic Bioethics Quarterly* 17, no. 1 (June 7, 2017): 43–49.

Babic, Boris, Sara Gerke, Theodoros Evgeniou, and I. Glenn Cohen. "Beware Explanations from AI in Health Care." *Science* 373, no. 6552 (July 16, 2021): 284–86. https://doi.org/10.1126/science.abg1834.

Badal, Varsha D., Sarah A. Graham, Colin A. Depp, Kaoru Shinkawa, Yasunori Yamada, Lawrence A. Palinkas, Ho-Cheol Kim, Dilip V. Jeste, and Ellen E. Lee.

"Prediction of Loneliness in Older Adults Using Natural Language Processing: Exploring Sex Differences in Speech." *American Journal of Geriatric Psychiatry* 29, no. 8 (August 1, 2021): 853–66. https://doi.org/10.1016/j.jagp.2020.09.009.

Barilan, Yechiel Michael. *Jewish Bioethics: Rabbinic Law and Theology in Their Social and Historical Contexts*. New York: Cambridge University Press, 2013.

Barina, Rachelle. "Prophylactic Salpingectomy to Reduce the Risk of Cancer." *Health Care Ethics USA* 23, no. 1 (2015): 31–33.

Barker, David. "The Biology of Stupidity: Genetics, Eugenics and Mental Deficiency in the Inter-war Years." *British Journal for the History of Science* 22, no. 3 (1989): 347–75.

Barnes, Elizabeth. *The Minority Body: A Theory of Disability*. Oxford: Oxford University Press, 2019.

Baylis, Françoise. *Altered Inheritance: CRISPR and the Ethics of Human Genome Editing*. Cambridge, MA: Harvard University Press, 2019.

Beck, Ulrich. *Risk Society*. London: Sage Publications, 1992.

———. *World at Risk*. New York: Polity Press, 2008.

Behforouz, Heidi L., Audrey Kalmus, China S. Scherz, Jeffrey S. Kahn, Mitul B. Kadakia, and Paul E. Farmer. "Directly Observed Therapy for HIV Antiretroviral Therapy in an Urban US Setting." *JAIDS: Journal of Acquired Immune Deficiency Syndromes* 36, no. 1 (May 1, 2004): 642–45.

Bell, Steven, Mika Kivimäki, and G. David Batty. "Subgroup Analysis as a Source of Spurious Findings: An Illustration Using New Data on Alcohol Intake and Coronary Heart Disease." *Addiction* 110, no. 1 (2015): 183–84. https://doi.org/10.1111/add.12708.

Belluck, Pam, Sheila Kaplan, and Rebecca Robbins. "How an Unproven Alzheimer's Drug Got Approved." *New York Times*, July 20, 2021, sec. Health. www.nytimes.com/2021/07/19/health/alzheimers-drug-aduhelm-fda.html.

Benedict. *Rule of Saint Benedict*. Translated by Bruce Venarde. Dumbarton Oaks Medieval Library 6. Cambridge, MA: Harvard University Press, 2011.

Benton, Adia. *HIV Exceptionalism: Development through Disease in Sierra Leone*. Minneapolis: University of Minnesota Press, 2015.

Berkman, John, and Robyn Boeré. "St. Thomas Aquinas on Impairment, Natural Goods, and Human Flourishing." *National Catholic Bioethics Quarterly* 20, no. 2 (October 21, 2020): 311–28.

Berkovich, Barbara, and Amy Sitipati. *Applied Population Health*. New York: CRC Press, 2020.

Bernstein, Peter. *Against the Gods: The Remarkable Story of Risk*. New York: Wiley, 1998.

Berwick, Donald M. "Health Services Research, Medicare, and Medicaid: A Deep Bow and a Rechartered Agenda." *Milbank Quarterly* 93, no. 4 (2015): 659–62.

———. "Making Good on ACOs' Promise: The Final Rule for the Medicare Shared Savings Program." *New England Journal of Medicine* 365, no. 19 (November 10, 2011): 1753–56. https://doi.org/10.1056/NEJMp1111671.

Berwick, Donald M., Thomas Nolan, and John Whittington. "The Triple Aim: Care, Health, and Cost." *Health Affairs* 27, no. 3 (2008): 759–69.

Bishop, Jeffrey Paul. *The Anticipatory Corpse: Medicine, Power, and the Care of the Dying*. Notre Dame, IN: University of Notre Dame Press, 2011.

Boltanski, Luc. *Distant Suffering: Morality, Media and Politics*. Translated by Graham D. Burchell. Cambridge: Cambridge University Press, 1999.

Boorse, Christopher. "Health as a Theoretical Concept." *Philosophy of Science* 44, no. 4 (1977): 542–73. https://doi.org/10.2307/186939.

Bosma, H., R. Peter, J. Siegrist, and M. Marmot. "Two Alternative Job Stress Models and the Risk of Coronary Heart Disease." *American Journal of Public Health* 88, no. 1 (January 1998): 68–74.

Bostrom, Nick. "Why I Want to Be a Posthuman When I Grow Up." In *The Transhumanist Reader*, edited by Max More and Natasha Vita-More, 28–53. Malden, MA: Wiley-Blackwell, 2013.

Bouk, Dan. *How Our Days Became Numbered: Risk and the Rise of the Statistical Individual*. Chicago: University of Chicago Press, 2015.

Bourdieu, Pierre. *Distinction: A Social Critique of the Judgement of Taste*. Cambridge, MA: Harvard University Press, 1984.

Bowler, Peter J. *The Mendelian Revolution: The Emergence of Hereditarian Concepts in Modern Science and Society*. Baltimore: Johns Hopkins University Press, 1989.

Braswell, Harold. *The Crisis of US Hospice Care*. Baltimore: Johns Hopkins University Press, 2019.

Breastcancer.org. "Breast Cancer Facts and Statistics." Accessed September 21, 2022. www.breastcancer.org/facts-statistics.

Bretthauer, Michael, Magnus Løberg, Paulina Wieszczy, Mette Kalager, Louise Emilsson, Kjetil Garborg, Maciej Rupinski, et al. "Effect of Colonoscopy Screening on Risks of Colorectal Cancer and Related Death." *New England Journal of Medicine* 387, no. 17 (October 27, 2022): 1547–56. https://doi.org/10.1056/NEJMoa2208375.

Brock, Dan. "Ethical Issues in the Use of Cost Effectiveness Analysis for the Prioritisation of Health Care Resources." In *Public Health, Ethics, and Equity*, edited by Sudhir Anand, Fabienne Peter, and Amartya Sen, 200–224. Oxford: Oxford University Press, 2004.

———. "Identified versus Statistical Lives: Some Introductory Issues and Arguments." In *Identified versus Statistical Lives: An Interdisciplinary Perspective*, edited by I. Glenn Cohen, Norman Daniels, and Nir M. Eyal, 43–52. Oxford: Oxford University Press, 2015.

Brown, Peter. *The Body and Society: Men, Women, and Sexual Renunciation in Early Christianity*. New York: Columbia University Press, 1988.
Burleigh, Michael. *Death and Deliverance: "Euthanasia" in Germany, c.1900 to 1945*. Cambridge: Cambridge University Press, 1995.
Butt, Leslie. "The Suffering Stranger: Medical Anthropology and International Morality." *Medical Anthropology* 21, no. 1 (2002): 1–24.
Bynum, Caroline Walker. *Fragmentation and Redemption: Essays on Gender and the Human Body in Medieval Religion*. New York: Zone Books, 1990.
Callahan, Daniel. *Setting Limits: Medical Goals in an Aging Society*. New York: Simon and Schuster, 1987.
Camosy, Charles. "Clearing Up the Catholic Confusion about Vaccine Mandates." *Religion News Service* (blog), August 13, 2021. https://religionnews.com/2021/08/13/clearing-up-the-catholic-confusion-about-vaccine-mandates/.
———. *Resisting Throwaway Culture: How a Consistent Life Ethic Can Unite a Fractured People*. Hyde Park, NY: New City Press, 2019.
———. *Too Expensive to Treat? Finitude, Tragedy, and the Neonatal ICU*. Grand Rapids, MI: Eerdmans, 2010.
Canguilhem, Georges. *The Normal and the Pathological*. New York: Zone Books, 1989.
Carlson, Elof. *The Unfit: A History of a Bad Idea*. Cold Spring Harbor, NY: Cold Spring Harbor Laboratory Press, 2001.
Carr, Nicholas. *The Glass Cage: How Computers Are Changing Us*. New York: Norton, 2015.
Cassell, Eric J. *The Nature of Suffering and the Goals of Medicine*. 2nd ed. New York: Oxford University Press, 2004.
Cassian, John. *The Conferences*. Translated by Boniface Ramsey. Ancient Christian Writers 57. New York: Paulist Press, 1997.
Cataldo, Peter. "Why the CDF 'Note on the Morality of Using Some Anti-Covid-19 Vaccines' Suggests a Moral Obligation to Receive SARS-CoV-2 Vaccines." *Health Care Ethics USA* 29, no. 4 (2021): 2–6.
Cayley, David, and Charles Taylor. *The Rivers North of the Future: The Testament of Ivan Illich*. New York: House of Anansi Press, 2005.
Centers for Disease Control. "Faststats: Leading Causes of Death." January 13, 2022. www.cdc.gov/nchs/fastats/leading-causes-of-death.htm.
———. "Leading Causes of Death, 1900–1998." www.cdc.gov/nchs/data/dvs/lead1900_98.pdf.
———. "Risk for COVID-19 Infection, Hospitalization, and Death by Age Group." Centers for Disease Control and Prevention, June 2, 2022. www.cdc.gov/coronavirus/2019-ncov/covid-data/investigations-discovery/hospitalization-death-by-age.html.

Charon, Rita. *Narrative Medicine: Honoring the Stories of Illness*. New York: Oxford University Press, 2008.

Childers, Timothy. *Philosophy and Probability*. New York: Oxford University Press, 2013.

Childress, James F., Ruth R. Faden, Ruth D. Gaare, Lawrence O. Gostin, Jeffrey Kahn, Richard J. Bonnie, Nancy E. Kass, Anna C. Mastroianni, Jonathan D. Moreno, and Phillip Nieburg. "Public Health Ethics: Mapping the Terrain." *Journal of Law, Medicine and Ethics* 30, no. 2 (2002): 170–78. https://doi.org/10.1111/j.1748-720x.2002.tb00384.x.

Clear, James. *Atomic Habits: An Easy and Proven Way to Build Good Habits and Break Bad Ones*. New York: Avery, 2018.

Clement of Alexandria. *Christ the Educator*. Translated by Simon Wood. The Fathers of the Church, vol. 23. Washington, DC: Catholic University of America Press, 1953.

Clinton, Bill, J. Craig Venter, James D. Watson, and Tony Blair. "Reading the Book of Life; White House Remarks on Decoding of Genome." *New York Times*, June 27, 2000. www.nytimes.com/2000/06/27/science/reading-the-book-of-life-white-house-remarks-on-decoding-of-genome.html.

Cloutier, David M. "The Workers' Paradise: Eternal Life, Economic Eschatology, and Good Work as the Keys to Social Ethics." *Proceedings of the Catholic Theological Society of America* 75 (January 1, 2021): 37–55.

Cloutier, David M., and William Mattison III. "The Resurgence of Virtue in Recent Moral Theology." *Journal of Moral Theology* 3, no. 1 (2014): 228–59.

Coblentz, Jessica. "Catholic Fasting Literature in a Context of Body Hatred: A Feminist Critique." *Horizons* 46, no. 2 (2019): 215–45. https://doi.org/10.1017/hor.2019.55.

Cohen, I. Glenn, Norman Daniels, and Nir M. Eyal, eds. *Identified versus Statistical Lives: An Interdisciplinary Perspective*. Oxford: Oxford University Press, 2015.

Cole-Turner, Ronald, ed. *Transhumanism and Transcendence: Christian Hope in an Age of Technological Enhancement*. Washington, DC: Georgetown University Press, 2011.

Collins, Francis S. *The Language of Life: DNA and the Revolution in Personalized Medicine*. New York: Harper Perennial, 2011.

Congregation for the Doctrine of the Faith. "Note on the Morality of Using Some Anti-Covid-19 Vaccines." December 21, 2020. www.vatican.va/roman_curia/congregations/cfaith/documents/rc_con_cfaith_doc_20201221_nota-vaccini-anticovid_en.html.

———. "Placuit Deo." January 3, 2018. https://press.vatican.va/content/salastampa/en/bollettino/pubblico/2018/03/01/180301a.html.

Coop, Graham, Michael B. Eisen, Rasmus Nielsen, Molly Przeworki, and Noah Rosenberg. "A Troublesome Inheritance." Letter to *New York Times Book Review*, August 8, 2014. https://cehg.stanford.edu/sites/g/files/sbiybj27086/files/media/file/letter-from-population-geneticists.pdf.

Craik, Elizabeth. *The "Hippocratic" Corpus: Content and Context*. New York: Routledge, 2014.

Crawford, Matthew B. *The World beyond Your Head: On Becoming an Individual in an Age of Distraction*. New York: Farrar, Straus and Giroux, 2016.

Crislip, Andrew. *From Monastery to Hospital: Christian Monasticism and the Transformation of Health Care in Late Antiquity*. Ann Arbor: University of Michigan Press, 2005.

Cronin, Daniel. *Ordinary and Extraordinary Means of Conserving Life*. 50th anniversary ed. Philadelphia: National Catholic Bioethics Center, 2011.

Cross, Ryan. "'Scientific Wellness' Study Divides Researchers." *Science* 357, no. 6349 (2017): 345.

Curlin, Farr. "Hospice and Palliative Medicine's Attempt at an Art of Dying." In *Dying in the Twenty-First Century: Toward a New Ethical Framework for the Art of Dying Well*, edited by Lydia Dugdale, 47–65. Cambridge, MA: MIT Press, 2016.

———. "'Sufficient for the Day Is Its Own Trouble': Medicalizing Risk and the Way of Jesus." *Christian Bioethics* 29, no. 2 (August 1, 2023): 110–19. https://doi.org/10.1093/cb/cbad014.

Cyprian. *Mortality*. In *Treatises*, edited and translated by Roy Deferrari, 199–221. The Fathers of the Church, vol. 36. Washington, DC: Catholic University of America Press, 1958.

Daniels, Norman. *Just Health Care*. Studies in Philosophy and Health Policy. Cambridge: Cambridge University Press, 1985.

Davis, Joseph E. "The Devalued Status of Old Age." In *The Evening of Life: The Challenges of Aging and Dying Well*, edited by Joseph E. Davis and Paul Scherz, 23–37. Notre Dame, IN: University of Notre Dame Press, 2020.

Davis, Joseph E., and Paul Scherz, eds. *The Evening of Life: The Challenges of Aging and Dying Well*. Notre Dame, IN: University of Notre Dame Press, 2020.

Dean, Mitchell. *Governmentality: Power and Rule in Modern Society*. Thousand Oaks, CA: Sage Publications, 1999.

Defert, Daniel. "'Popular Life' and Insurance Technology." In *The Foucault Effect*, edited by Graham Burchell, Colin Gordon, and Peter Miller. London: Harvester Wheatsheaf, 1991.

Desrosieres, Alain. *The Politics of Large Numbers*. Translated by Camille Naish. Cambridge, MA: Harvard University Press, 1998.

Dickenson, Donna. *Me Medicine vs. We Medicine: Reclaiming Biotechnology for the Common Good*. New York: Columbia University Press, 2013.

Dostoevsky, Fyodor. *Notes from Underground*. Translated by Michael Katz. New York: Norton, 1989.

Doudna, Jennifer A., and Samuel H. Sternberg. *A Crack in Creation: Gene Editing and the Unthinkable Power to Control Evolution*. Boston: Mariner Books, 2018.

Droge, Mitchell. "What Is Quantified Self?" *Quantified Self Institute* (blog), October 18, 2016. http://qsinstitute.com/about/what-is-quantified-self/.

Dumit, Joseph. *Drugs for Life: How Pharmaceutical Companies Define Our Health*. Durham, NC: Duke University Press, 2012.

Dworkin, Ronald W. *Medical Catastrophe: Confessions of an Anesthesiologist*. Lanham, MD: Rowman and Littlefield, 2017.

Eberl, Jason T. "Is There a Moral Obligation to Be Vaccinated for COVID-19?" *Health Care Ethics USA* 30, no. 1 (2022): 33–39.

———. "A Thomistic Appraisal of Human Enhancement Technologies." *Theoretical Medicine and Bioethics* 35, no. 4 (August 2014): 289–310. https://doi.org/10.1007/s11017-014-9300-x.

Eberl, Jason T., and Tobias Winright. "Catholics Have No Grounds to Claim Exemption from COVID Vaccine Mandates." *National Catholic Reporter*, August 27, 2021. www.ncronline.org/news/coronavirus/catholics-have-no-grounds-claim-exemption-covid-vaccine-mandates.

Edelstein, Ludwig. "The Dietetics of Antiquity." In *Ancient Medicine: Selected Papers of Ludwig Edelstein*, 303–16. Baltimore: Johns Hopkins University Press, 1987.

Ehrenreich, Barbara. *Natural Causes*. New York: Twelve, 2018.

Elliott, Carl. "Why Clinical Ethicists Are Not Activists." *Hastings Center Report* 51, no. 4 (2021): 36–37. https://doi.org/10.1002/hast.1272.

Emanuel, Ezekiel, Govind Persad, Ross Upshur, Beatriz Thome, Michael Parker, Aaron Glickman, Cathy Zhang, et al. "Fair Allocation of Scarce Medical Resources in the Time of Covid-19." *New England Journal of Medicine* 382 (2020): 2049–55.

Enos, William F., Jr., James C. Beyer, and Robert H. Holmes. "Pathogenesis of Coronary Disease in American Soldiers Killed in Korea." *Journal of the American Medical Association* 158, no. 11 (July 16, 1955): 912–14. https://doi.org/10.1001/jama.1955.02960110018005.

Epstein, Helen. *The Invisible Cure: Why We Are Losing the Fight against AIDS in Africa*. New York: Picador, 2008.

Evans, John H. *Playing God? Human Genetic Engineering and the Rationalization of Public Bioethical Debate*. Chicago: University of Chicago Press, 2002.

Ewald, Francois. *The Birth of Solidarity: The History of the French Welfare State*. Translated by Timothy Scott Johnson. Durham, NC: Duke University Press, 2020.

———. *L'état Providence*. Paris: Grasset, 1986.

Farmer, Paul. "Chronic Infectious Disease and the Future of Health Care Delivery." *New England Journal of Medicine* 369, no. 25 (December 19, 2013): 2424–36. https://doi.org/10.1056/NEJMsa1310472.

———. *Pathologies of Power: Health, Human Rights, and the New War on the Poor.* Berkeley: University of California Press, 2004.

Ferngren, Gary B. *Medicine and Health Care in Early Christianity.* Baltimore: Johns Hopkins University Press, 2009.

Ferrie, J. E., M. J. Shipley, M. G. Marmot, S. A. Stansfeld, and G. D. Smith. "An Uncertain Future: The Health Effects of Threats to Employment Security in White-Collar Men and Women." *American Journal of Public Health* 88, no. 7 (July 1998): 1030–36.

Feuerstein, Adam. "Bluebird's Withdrawal of Therapy from Germany Could Chill Talks over Gene Therapy Prices across Europe." *STAT* (blog), April 22, 2021. www.statnews.com/2021/04/22/bluebirds-withdrawal-of-therapy-from-germany-could-chill-talks-over-gene-therapy-prices-across-europe/.

Finkelstein, Amy, Annetta Zhou, Sarah Taubman, and Joseph Doyle. "Health Care Hotspotting: A Randomized, Controlled Trial." *New England Journal of Medicine* 382, no. 2 (January 9, 2020): 152–62. https://doi.org/10.1056/NEJMsa1906848.

Finnis, John. "Practical Reasoning, Human Goods and the End of Man." *New Blackfriars* 66, no. 784 (October 1, 1985): 438–51.

Fisher, Irving, and Eugene Fisk. *How to Live: Rules for Healthful Living Based on Modern Science.* 16th ed. New York: Funk and Wagnalls, 1922.

Foot, Philippa. *Natural Goodness.* Oxford: Clarendon Press, 2003.

Fortun, Mike. *Promising Genomics.* Berkeley: University of California Press, 2008.

Foucault, Michel. *The Birth of Biopolitics: Lectures at the Collège de France, 1978–79.* Edited by Michel Senellart. New York: Palgrave Macmillan, 2008.

———. *The Care of the Self.* New York: Pantheon Books, 1986.

———. *The Courage of Truth: The Government of Self and Others II: Lectures at the Collège de France, 1983–1984.* Translated by Graham Burchell. New York: Palgrave Macmillan, 2011.

———. *Discipline and Punish: The Birth of the Prison.* New York: Pantheon Books, 1977.

———. *The Hermeneutics of the Subject: Lectures at the Collège de France, 1981–82.* Translated by Graham Burchell. New York: Palgrave Macmillan, 2005.

———. *History of Madness.* Translated by Jonathan Murphy. New York: Routledge, 2006.

———. *The History of Sexuality.* Vol 1. New York: Pantheon Books, 1978.

———. *Security, Territory, Population: Lectures at the Collège de France, 1977–78.* Edited by Michel Senellart. Translated by Graham Burchell. New York: Palgrave Macmillan, 2007.

———. *Society Must Be Defended: Lectures at the Collège de France, 1975–76.* Edited by Mauro Bertani and Alessandro Fontana. Translated by David Macey. New York: Picador, 2003.

———. *The Use of Pleasure.* New York: Vintage Books, 1985.

Foucault, Michel, Graham Burchell, Colin Gordon, and Peter Miller. *The Foucault Effect: Studies in Governmentality.* Chicago: University of Chicago Press, 1991.

Francis. "Moment of Prayer and 'Urbi et Orbi' Blessing." March 27, 2020. www.vatican.va/content/francesco/en/homilies/2020/documents/papa francesco _20200327_omelia-epidemia.html.

Fried, Charles. "The Value of Life." *Harvard Law Review* 82, no. 7 (1969): 1415–37.

Gadamer, Hans-Georg. *The Enigma of Health.* Stanford, CA: Stanford University Press, 1996.

Gane, Mike. "Foucault on Governmentality and Liberalism." *Theory, Culture and Society* 25, no. 7–8 (2008): 353–63.

Gawande, Atul. *Being Mortal: Medicine and What Matters in the End.* New York: Metropolitan Books, 2014.

———. "The Hot Spotters." *New Yorker*, January 24, 2011.

———. "Whose Body Is It, Anyway?" *New Yorker*, October 4, 1999.

"Gene Therapies Should Be for All." *Nature Medicine* 27, no. 8 (August 2021): 1311. https://doi.org/10.1038/s41591-021-01481-9.

Gibson, Greg. "On the Utilization of Polygenic Risk Scores for Therapeutic Targeting." *PLOS Genetics* 15, no. 4 (April 2019): e1008060. https://doi.org/10.1371/journal.pgen.1008060.

Gigerenzer, Gerd. *Rationality for Mortals.* New York: Oxford University Press, 2008.

Gillespie, Chris. "The Experience of Risk as 'Measured Vulnerability': Health Screening and Lay Uses of Numerical Risk." *Sociology of Health and Illness* 34, no. 2 (2012): 194–207. https://doi.org/10.1111/j.1467-9566.2011.01381.x.

Goffman, Erving. *Asylums: Essays on the Social Situation of Mental Patients and Other Inmates.* Garden City, NY: Anchor Books, 1961.

Goldstone, Brian. "A Prayer's Chance." *Harper's* magazine, May 1, 2017. https://harpers.org/archive/2017/05/a-prayers-chance/.

Gould, Stephen Jay. "The Median Isn't the Message." In *Bully for Brontosaurus: Reflections in Natural History*, 473–78. New York: Norton, 1991.

———. *The Mismeasure of Man.* 2nd ed. New York: Norton, 1996.

Graeber, David. *Bullshit Jobs: A Theory.* New York: Simon and Schuster, 2018.

Greely, Henry T. *CRISPR People: The Science and Ethics of Editing Humans.* Cambridge, MA: MIT Press, 2021.

Greene, Jeremy A. *Prescribing by Numbers: Drugs and the Definition of Disease.* Baltimore: Johns Hopkins University Press, 2008.

Gregory, Bradley C. "The Tree of Life, Health, and Risk through the Lens of Biblical Wisdom." *Christian Bioethics: Non-ecumenical Studies in Medical Morality* 29, no. 2 (August 1, 2023): 129–40. https://doi.org/10.1093/cb/cbad009.

Grisez, Germain. "The First Principle of Practical Reason: A Commentary on the Summa Theologiae, 1-2, Question 94, Article 2." *American Journal of Jurisprudence* 10, no. 1 (January 1, 1965): 168–201.

———. "Should Nutrition and Hydration Be Provided to Permanently Unconscious and Other Mentally Disabled Persons?" *Issues in Law and Medicine* 5, no. 2 (1989): 165–79.

Grob, Rachel. *Testing Baby: The Transformation of Newborn Screening, Parenting, and Policymaking*. New Brunswick, NJ: Rutgers University Press, 2011.

Gyawali, Bishal, Richard Sullivan, and Christopher M. Booth. "Cancer Groundshot: Going Global before Going to the Moon." *Lancet Oncology* 19, no. 3 (March 1, 2018): 288–90. https://doi.org/10.1016/S1470-2045(18)30076-7.

Habib, Anand R., Mitchell H. Katz, and Rita F. Redberg. "Statins for Primary Cardiovascular Disease Prevention: Time to Curb Our Enthusiasm." *JAMA Internal Medicine* 182, no. 10 (October 1, 2022): 1021–24. https://doi.org/10.1001/jamainternmed.2022.3204.

Hacking, Ian. *The Taming of Chance*. Cambridge: Cambridge University Press, 1990.

Hadler, Nortin M. *By the Bedside of the Patient: Lessons for the Twenty-First-Century Physician*. Chapel Hill, NC: University of North Carolina Press, 2016.

———. *The Last Well Person: How to Stay Well Despite the Health-Care System*. Montreal: McGill-Queen's University Press, 2007.

———. *Worried Sick: A Prescription for Health in an Overtreated America*. Chapel Hill: University of North Carolina Press, 2012.

Hadot, Pierre. *Philosophy as a Way of Life: Spiritual Exercises from Socrates to Foucault*. Translated by Arnold I. Davidson. Cambridge, MA: Blackwell, 1995.

Hamel, Ronald P. "Catholic Identity, Ethics Need Focus in New Era." *Health Progress* 94, no. 3 (June 2013): 85–87.

Hamel, Ronald P., and James J. Walter, eds. *Artificial Nutrition and Hydration and the Permanently Unconscious Patient: The Catholic Debate*. Washington, DC: Georgetown University Press, 2007.

Harden, Kathryn Paige. *The Genetic Lottery: Why DNA Matters for Social Equity*. Princeton, NJ: Princeton University Press, 2021.

Harris, John. *Enhancing Evolution: The Ethical Case for Making Better People*. Princeton, NJ: Princeton University Press, 2007.

Haslam, Alyson, Timothée Olivier, Jordan Tuia, and Vinay Prasad. "Umbrella Review of Basket Trials Testing a Drug in Tumors with Actionable Genetic Biomarkers." *BMC Cancer* 23, no. 1 (January 13, 2023): 46. https://doi.org/10.1186/s12885-022-10421-w.

Hauerwas, Stanley. *Suffering Presence: Theological Reflections on Medicine, the Mentally Handicapped, and the Church*. Notre Dame, IN: University of Notre Dame Press, 1986.

Head, Jenny, Mika Kivimäki, Pekka Martikainen, Jussi Vahtera, Jane E. Ferrie, and Michael G. Marmot. "Influence of Change in Psychosocial Work Characteristics on Sickness Absence: The Whitehall II Study." *Journal of Epidemiology and Community Health* 60, no. 1 (January 2006): 55–61. https://doi.org/10.1136/jech.2005.038752.

Heidegger, Martin. *Being and Time*. Translated by John Macquarrie and Edward Robinson. New York: HarperCollins, 2008.

Herrnstein, Richard, and Charles Murray. *The Bell Curve*. New York: Free Press, 1996.

Hey, Spencer Phillips, Cory V. Gerlach, Garrett Dunlap, Vinay Prasad, and Aaron S. Kesselheim. "The Evidence Landscape in Precision Medicine." *Science Translational Medicine* 12, no. 540 (April 22, 2020): eaaw7745. https://doi.org/10.1126/scitranslmed.aaw7745.

Hittinger, Russell. "The Coherence of the Four Basic Principles of Catholic Social Doctrine: An Interpretation." *Nova et Vetera* 7, no. 4 (2009): 791–838.

Hochman, Rod, and Sr. Donna Markham, O.P. "Love and Logic: Catholic Health Care and Catholic Charities Bring Expertise and Robust Partnership Possibilities." *Health Progress* 99, no. 5 (October 2018): 19–21.

Hou, Ying-Chen Claire, Hung-Chun Yu, Rick Martin, Elizabeth T. Cirulli, Natalie M. Schenker-Ahmed, Michael Hicks, Isaac V. Cohen, et al. "Precision Medicine Integrating Whole-Genome Sequencing, Comprehensive Metabolomics, and Advanced Imaging." *Proceedings of the National Academy of Sciences* 117, no. 6 (February 11, 2020): 3053–62. https://doi.org/10.1073/pnas.1909378117.

Hudson, Kathy L., and Karen Pollitz. "Undermining Genetic Privacy? Employee Wellness Programs and the Law." *New England Journal of Medicine* 377, no. 1 (July 6, 2017): 1–3.

Hursthouse, Rosalind. *On Virtue Ethics*. Oxford: Oxford University Press, 2002.

Illich, Ivan. *Deschooling Society*. New York: Harper and Row, 1971.

———. *Limits to Medicine: Medical Nemesis, the Expropriation of Health*. London: Marion Boyars, 2016.

Illich, Ivan, Irving K. Zola, and John McKnight. *Disabling Professions*. New York: Marion Boyars, 2000.

Institute for Human Ecology. "The COVID Vaccine: Science, Life and the Common Good." Panel discussion, Institute for Human Ecology, January 14, 2021. https://ihe.catholic.edu/event/the-covid-vaccine-science-life-and-the-common-good/.

Ioannidis, John P. A., Michael E. Stuart, Shannon Brownlee, and Sheri A. Strite. "How to Survive the Medical Misinformation Mess." *European Journal of Clinical Investigation* 47 (2017): 795–802. https://doi.org/10.1111/eci.12834.

Iovan, Samantha, Paula M. Lantz, Katie Allan, and Mahshid Abir. "Interventions to Decrease Use in Prehospital and Emergency Care Settings among Super-utilizers in the United States: A Systematic Review." *Medical Care Research and Review: MCRR* 77, no. 2 (April 2020): 99–111. https://doi.org/10.1177/1077558719845722.

Jahn, Jaquelyn L., Edward L. Giovannucci, and Meir J. Stampfer. "The High Prevalence of Undiagnosed Prostate Cancer at Autopsy: Implications for Epidemiology and Treatment of Prostate Cancer in the Prostate-Specific Antigen-Era." *International Journal of Cancer* 137, no. 12 (December 15, 2015): 2795–2802. https://doi.org/10.1002/ijc.29408.

James, Jennifer Elyse, Leslie Riddle, Barbara Ann Koenig, and Galen Joseph. "The Limits of Personalization in Precision Medicine: Polygenic Risk Scores and Racial Categorization in a Precision Breast Cancer Screening Trial." *PLOS One* 16, no. 10 (2021): e0258571. https://doi.org/10.1371/journal.pone.0258571.

Jensen, Arthur. "How Much Can We Boost I.Q. and Scholastic Achievement?" *Harvard Educational Review* 33 (1969): 1–123.

John Paul II. *Evangelium Vitae*. March 25, 1995. www.vatican.va/content/john-paul-ii/en/encyclicals/documents/hf_jp-ii_enc_25031995_evangelium-vitae.html.

———. *Man and Woman He Created Them: A Theology of the Body*. Translated by Michael Waldstein. Boston: Pauline Books and Media, 2006.

———. *Sollicitudo Rei Socialis*. December 30, 1987. www.vatican.va/content/john-paul-ii/en/encyclicals/documents/hf_jp-ii_enc_30121987_sollicitudo-rei-socialis.html.

Johnston, Josephine, John D. Lantos, Aaron Goldenberg, Flavia Chen, Erik Parens, Barbara A. Koenig, and members of the NSIGHT Ethics and Policy Advisory Board. "Sequencing Newborns: A Call for Nuanced Use of Genomic Technologies." *Hastings Center Report* 48, no. S2 (2018): S2–6. https://doi.org/10.1002/hast.874.

Jonas, Hans. *The Gnostic Religion: The Message of the Alien God and the Beginnings of Christianity*. Boston: Beacon Press, 1958.

Jonsen, Albert. "Bentham in a Box: Technology Assessment and Health Care Allocation." *Law, Medicine and Health Care* 14, nos. 3–4 (1986): 172–74.

———. *The Birth of Bioethics*. Oxford: Oxford University Press, 2003.

"Judge Blocks New York City Large-Soda Ban, Mayor Bloomberg Vows Fight." Reuters, March 11, 2013, sec. Healthcare & Pharma. www.reuters.com/article/us-sodaban-lawsuit-idUSBRE92A0YR20130311.

Judson, Horace Freeland. *The Eighth Day of Creation: Makers of the Revolution in Biology*. Plainview, NY: Cold Spring Harbor Laboratory Press, 1996.
Juengst, Eric, Michelle L. McGowan, Jennifer R. Fishman, and Richard A. Settersten. "From 'Personalized' to 'Precision' Medicine: The Ethical and Social Implications of Rhetorical Reform in Genomic Medicine." *Hastings Center Report* 46, no. 5 (September 2016): 21–33. https://doi.org/10.1002/hast.614.
Kahn, Jeffrey, and Anna Mastroianni. "The Implications of Public Health for Bioethics." In *The Oxford Handbook of Bioethics*, edited by Bonnie Steinbock, 671–95. Oxford: Oxford University Press, 2009. https://doi.org/10.1093/oxfordhb/9780199562411.003.0029.
Kahneman, Daniel. *Thinking, Fast and Slow*. New York: Farrar, Straus and Giroux, 2013.
Kaplan, Jonathan Michael, and Stephanie M. Fullerton. "Polygenic Risk, Population Structure and Ongoing Difficulties with Race in Human Genetics." *Philosophical Transactions of the Royal Society of London. Series B, Biological Sciences* 377, no. 1852 (June 6, 2022): 20200427. https://doi.org/10.1098/rstb.2020.0427.
Kass, Leon. *Life, Liberty, and the Defense of Dignity*. San Francisco: Encounter, 2002.
Kaufman, Sharon R. *And a Time to Die: How American Hospitals Shape the End of Life*. Chicago: University of Chicago Press, 2006.
———. *Ordinary Medicine: Extraordinary Treatments, Longer Lives, and Where to Draw the Line*. Durham, NC: Duke University Press, 2015.
Kavin Rowe, C. "Theology, Medicalization, and Risk: Observations from the New Testament." *Christian Bioethics: Non-ecumenical Studies in Medical Morality* 29, no. 2 (August 1, 2023): 120–28. https://doi.org/10.1093/cb/cbad008.
Kay, Lily. *The Molecular Vision of Life: Caltech, the Rockefeller Foundation, and the Rise of the New Biology*. New York: Oxford University Press, 1996.
———. *Who Wrote the Book of Life? A History of the Genetic Code*. Stanford, CA: Stanford University Press, 2000.
Kaye, Howard. *The Social Meaning of Modern Biology*. New Haven, CT: Yale University Press, 1986.
Keane, Philip S. *Catholicism and Health-Care Justice: Problems, Potential and Solutions*. New York: Paulist Press, 2002.
Kell, Douglas B., and Stephen G. Oliver. "Here Is the Evidence, Now What Is the Hypothesis? The Complementary Roles of Inductive and Hypothesis-Driven Science in the Post-Genomic Era." *BioEssays: News and Reviews in Molecular, Cellular and Developmental Biology* 26, no. 1 (January 2004): 99–105. https://doi.org/10.1002/bies.10385.
Kelly, Conor. "On Pediatric Vaccines and Catholic Social Teaching." *Horizons* 45, no. 2 (2018): 287–316.

Kelly, Gerald. "The Duty of Using Artificial Means of Preserving Life." *Theological Studies* 11, no. 2 (May 1, 1950): 203–20. https://doi.org/10.1177/004056395001100202.

———. "The Duty to Preserve Life." *Theological Studies* 12, no. 4 (December 1, 1951): 550–56. https://doi.org/10.1177/004056395101200405.

Kevles, Daniel. *In the Name of Eugenics: Genetics and the Uses of Human Heredity*. Cambridge, MA: Harvard University Press, 1995.

Kheriaty, Aaron. *The New Abnormal: The Rise of the Biomedical Security State*. Washington, DC: Regnery, 2022.

Kidder, Tracy. *Mountains beyond Mountains: The Quest of Dr. Paul Farmer, a Man Who Would Cure the World*. New York: Random House, 2009.

Kinghorn, Warren. "Protecting Life or Managing Risk? Suicide Prevention and the Lure of Medicalized Control." *Christian Bioethics* 29, no. 2 (August 1, 2023): 152–63. https://doi.org/10.1093/cb/cbad010.

Kittay, Eva Feder. "We Have Seen the Mutants—and They Are Us: Gifts and Burdens of a Genetic Diagnosis." *Hastings Center Report* 50, no. S1 (2020): S44–53. https://doi.org/10.1002/hast.1155.

Kivimäki, Mika, Solja T. Nyberg, Jaana Pentti, Ida E. H. Madsen, Linda L. Magnusson Hanson, Reiner Rugulies, Jussi Vahtera, David Coggon, and IPD-Work Consortium. "Individual and Combined Effects of Job Strain Components on Subsequent Morbidity and Mortality." *Epidemiology* 30, no. 4 (July 2019): e27–29. https://doi.org/10.1097/EDE.0000000000001020.

Klibansky, Raymond, Erwin Panofsky, and Fritz Saxl. *Saturn and Melancholy: Studies in the History of Natural Philosophy, Religion, and Art*. London: Nelson and Sons, 1964.

Knight, Frank H. *Risk, Uncertainty and Profit*. Ithaca, NY: Cornell University Library, 2009.

Krieger, Nancy. "Who and What Is a 'Population'? Historical Debates, Current Controversies, and Implications for Understanding 'Population Health' and Rectifying Health Inequities." *Milbank Quarterly* 90, no. 4 (December 2012): 634–81. https://doi.org/10.1111/j.1468-0009.2012.00678.x.

Krogsbøll, Lasse, Karsten Jørgensen, and Peter Gøtzsche. "General Health Checks in Adults for Reducing Morbidity and Mortality from Disease." *Cochrane Database of Systematic Reviews*, no. 1 (2019): CD009009.

Krugman, Paul. "An Insurance Company with an Army." *The Conscience of a Liberal* (blog), April 27, 2011. https://krugman.blogs.nytimes.com/2011/04/27/an-insurance-company-with-an-army/.

Kurzweil, Ray. *The Singularity Is Near*. New York: Viking, 2005.

Lander, Eric S. "The Heroes of CRISPR." *Cell* 164, nos. 1–2 (January 2016): 18–28. https://doi.org/10.1016/j.cell.2015.12.041.

Landry, Latrice G., Nadya Ali, David R. Williams, Heidi L. Rehm, and Vence L. Bonham. "Lack of Diversity in Genomic Databases Is a Barrier to Translating Precision Medicine Research into Practice." *Health Affairs* 37, no. 5 (May 2018): 780–85. https://doi.org/10.1377/hlthaff.2017.1595.

Lantz, Paula M. "The Medicalization of Population Health: Who Will Stay Upstream?" *Milbank Quarterly* 97, no. 1 (March 2019): 36–39. https://doi.org/10.1111/1468-0009.12363.

———. "'Super utilizer' Interventions: What They Reveal about Evaluation Research, Wishful Thinking, and Health Equity." *Milbank Quarterly* 98, no. 1 (March 2020): 31–34. https://doi.org/10.1111/1468-0009.12449.

László, Krisztina D., Hynek Pikhart, Mária S. Kopp, Martin Bobak, Andrzej Pajak, Sofia Malyutina, Gyöngyvér Salavecz, and Michael Marmot. "Job Insecurity and Health: A Study of 16 European Countries." *Social Science and Medicine* 70, no. 6–3 (March 2010): 867–74. https://doi.org/10.1016/j.socscimed.2009.11.022.

Leder, Drew. *The Absent Body*. Chicago: University of Chicago Press, 1990.

Leek, Jeff, Blakeley B. McShane, Andrew Gelman, David Colquhoun, Michèle B. Nuijten, and Steven N. Goodman. "Five Ways to Fix Statistics." *Nature* 551, no. 7682 (November 2017): 557–59. https://doi.org/10.1038/d41586-017-07522-z.

Leon, Sharon. *An Image of God*. Chicago: University of Chicago Press, 2013.

Lewis, Sinclair. *Arrowsmith*. New York: Harcourt Brace Jovanovich, 1952.

Lewontin, Richard. "The Apportionment of Human Diversity." *Evolutionary Biology* 6 (1972): 391–98.

———. *Biology as Ideology*. New York: Harper Perennial, 1991.

London, Alex. *For the Common Good: Philosophical Foundations of Research Ethics*. New York: Oxford University Press, 2021.

Löwy, Ilana. *Preventive Strikes: Women, Precancer, and Prophylactic Surgery*. Baltimore: Johns Hopkins University Press, 2009.

Luhmann, Niklas. *Risk: A Sociological Theory*. Translated by Rhodes Barrett. New Brunswick, NJ: Aldine Transaction, 2005.

Lundh, Andreas, Sergio Sismondo, Joel Lexchin, Octavian A. Busuioc, and Lisa Bero. "Industry Sponsorship and Research Outcome." *Cochrane Database of Systematic Reviews* 12 (December 12, 2012): MR000033. https://doi.org/10.1002/14651858.MR000033.pub2.

Lupton, Deborah. *The Imperative of Health: Public Health and the Regulated Body*. London: Sage Publications, 1995.

———. *The Quantified Self*. New York: Polity Press, 2016.

Lustig, B. Andrew. "Reform and Rationing: Reflections on Health Care in Light of Catholic Social Teaching." In *On Moral Medicine*, edited by M. Therese Lysaught, Joseph Kotva, Stephen Lammers, and Allen Verhey, 3rd ed., 201–10. Grand Rapids, MI: Eerdmans, 2012.

Lysaught, M. Therese. "Catholics Seeking 'Religious' Exemptions to Vaccines Must Follow True Church Teaching on Conscience." *National Catholic Reporter*, September 21, 2021. www.ncronline.org/news/opinion/catholics-seeking-religious-exemptions-vaccines-must-follow-true-church-teaching.

MacIntyre, Alasdair. *After Virtue: A Study in Moral Theory*. 2nd ed. Notre Dame, IN: University of Notre Dame Press, 1984.

MacKenzie, Donald. *Statistics in Britain, 1965–1930: The Social Construction of Scientific Knowledge*. Edinburgh: Edinburgh University Press, 1981.

MacKenzie, Donald, and Barry Barnes. "Scientific Judgment: The Biometry-Mendelism Controversy." In *Natural Order: Historical Studies of Scientific Culture*, edited by Barry Barnes and Steven Shapin, 191–210. London: Sage Publications, 1979.

Macrobius, Ambrosius Aurelius Theodosius. *Commentary on the Dream of Scipio*. New York: Columbia University Press, 1990.

Mandrola, John, and Vinay Prasad. "Screening Colonoscopy Misses the Mark in Its First Real Test." *Sensible Medicine*, October 10, 2022. https://sensiblemed.substack.com/p/screening-colonoscopy-misses-the?publication_id=1000397&isFreemail=true.

Mapes, Brandy M., Christopher S. Foster, Sheila V. Kusnoor, Marcia I. Epelbaum, Mona AuYoung, Gwynne Jenkins, Maria Lopez-Class, et al. "Diversity and Inclusion for the All of Us Research Program: A Scoping Review." *PLOS One* 15, no. 7 (2020): e0234962. https://doi.org/10.1371/journal.pone.0234962.

Marks, Jonathan. *Is Science Racist?* Cambridge: Polity Press, 2017.

Marmot, Michael. *The Health Gap*. London: Bloomsbury, 2016.

———. "Social Determinants of Health Inequalities." *Lancet* 365 (2005): 1099–1104.

———. *The Status Syndrome: How Social Standing Affects Our Health and Longevity*. New York: Owl Books, 2005.

Marseille, Elliot, Paul B. Hofmann, and James G. Kahn. "HIV Prevention before HAART in Sub-Saharan Africa." *The Lancet* 359, no. 9320 (May 25, 2002): 1851–56. https://doi.org/10.1016/S0140-6736(02)08705-6.

Mathieson, Iain, and Aylwyn Scally. "What Is Ancestry?" *PLOS Genetics* 16, no. 3 (March 9, 2020): e1008624. https://doi.org/10.1371/journal.pgen.1008624.

Mattison, William C., III. *Growing in Virtue: Aquinas on Habit*. Washington, DC: Georgetown University Press, 2023.

McKenny, Gerald. *Biotechnology, Human Nature, and Christian Ethics*. New Studies in Christian Ethics. New York: Cambridge University Press, 2018.

———. *To Relieve the Human Condition: Bioethics, Technology, and the Body*. Albany, NY: State University of New York Press, 1997.

McKeown, Thomas. *The Modern Rise of Population*. London: Edward Arnold, 1976.

McKinnon, Susan. *Neo-liberal Genetics*. Chicago: Prickly Paradigm Press, 2005.

McPhillips, Deidre. "FDA Approves $3.5 Million Treatment for Hemophilia, Now the Most Expensive Drug in the World." CNN, November 23, 2022. www.cnn.com/2022/11/23/health/hemophilia-drug-hemgenix/index.html.

Mescher, Marcus. *The Ethics of Encounter*. Maryknoll, NY: Orbis, 2020.

Messer, Neil. *Flourishing: Health, Disease, and Bioethics in Theological Perspective*. Grand Rapids, MI: Eerdmans, 2013.

Metzl, Jonathan M., and Anna Kirkland, eds. *Against Health. How Health Became the New Morality*. New York: NYU Press, 2010.

Miller, Stephen G., ed. *Arete: Greek Sports from Ancient Sources*. Berkeley: University of California Press, 1991.

Mitchell, Cory D., and M. Therese Lysaught. "Equally Strange Fruit: Catholic Health Care and the Appropriation of Residential Segregation." *Journal of Moral Theology* 8, no. 1 (January 1, 2019): 36–62.

Mjåset, Christer, Umar Ikram, Navraj Nagra, and Thomas Feeley. "Value-Based Health Care in Four Different Health Care Systems." *NEJM Catalyst Innovations in Care Delivery*, November 10, 2020. https://catalyst.nejm.org/doi/full/10.1056/CAT.20.0530.

Mol, Annemarie. *The Logic of Care: Health and the Problem of Patient Choice*. London: Routledge, 2008.

Mouloua, Mustapha, and R. Parasuraman. *Automation and Human Performance: Theory and Applications*. Human Factors in Transportation. Mahwah, NJ: Lawrence Erlbaum Associates, 1996.

Mounk, Yascha. *The Age of Responsibility: Luck, Choice, and the Welfare State*. Cambridge, MA: Harvard University Press, 2017.

Muller, Jerry. *The Tyranny of Metrics*. Princeton, NJ: Princeton University Press, 2018.

Müller-Wille, Staffan, and Hans-Jörg Rheinberger. *A Cultural History of Heredity*. Chicago: University of Chicago Press, 2012.

Mutter, Justin. "A New Stranger at the Bedside: Industrial Quality Management and the Erosion of Clinical Judgment in American Medicine." *Social Research* 86, no. 4 (2019): 931–54.

National Academies of Sciences, Engineering. *Statistical Challenges in Assessing and Fostering the Reproducibility of Scientific Results: Summary of a Workshop*. Washington, DC: National Academies Press, 2016. https://doi.org/10.17226/21915.

National Cancer Institute. "BRCA Gene Mutations: Cancer Risk and Genetic Testing Fact Sheet." November 25, 2020. www.cancer.gov/about-cancer/causes-prevention/genetics/brca-fact-sheet.

———. "Cancer Moonshot[SM]." February 1, 2016. www.cancer.gov/research/key-initiatives/moonshot-cancer-initiative.

National Center for Health Statistics. *Health, United States, 2016: With Chartbook on Long-Term Trends in Health*. Hyattsville, MD: US Government Printing Office, 2017.

National Health Service. "Getting a COVID-19 Vaccine." March 20, 2023. www.nhs.uk/conditions/covid-19/covid-19-vaccination/getting-a-covid-19-vaccine/.

National Human Genome Research Institute. "Genetic Discrimination." Accessed May 31, 2022. www.genome.gov/about-genomics/policy-issues/Genetic-Discrimination.

National Institute for Health and Care Excellence. "Prostate Cancer: Diagnosis and Management. Recommendations." May 9, 2019. www.nice.org.uk/guidance/ng131/chapter/Recommendations#assessment-and-diagnosis.

Nelkin, Dorothy, and M. Susan Lindee. *The DNA Mystique: The Gene as a Cultural Icon*. Ann Arbor: University of Michigan Press, 2004.

Nelson, Alondra. *The Social Life of DNA: Race, Reparations, and Reconciliation after the Genome*. Boston: Beacon Press, 2016.

Nogrady, Bianca. "How Cancer Genomics Is Transforming Diagnosis and Treatment." *Nature* 579, no. 7800 (March 25, 2020): S10–11. https://doi.org/10.1038/d41586-020-00845-4.

Nordenfelt, L. Y. *On the Nature of Health: An Action-Theoretic Approach*. Dordrecht: Springer, 2013.

Nuijten, Michèle B. "Practical Tools and Strategies for Researchers to Increase Replicability." *Developmental Medicine and Child Neurology* 61, no. 5 (2019): 535–39. https://doi.org/10.1111/dmcn.14054.

Nutton, Vivian. *Ancient Medicine*. 2nd ed. London: Routledge, 2012.

O'Callaghan, Tiffany. "Mammogram Recommendations Spark Controversy, Confusion." *Time*, November 17, 2009. https://healthland.time.com/2009/11/17/new-mammogram-recommendations-spark-controversy-and-confusion/.

Olby, Robert C. *Origins of Mendelism*. Chicago: University of Chicago Press, 1985.

O'Malley, Pat. "Governmentality and Risk." In *Social Theories of Risk and Uncertainty*, edited by Jens Zinn, 52–75. Malden, MA: Blackwell, 2008.

100,000 Genomes Project Pilot Investigators. "100,000 Genomes Pilot on Rare-Disease Diagnosis in Health Care." *New England Journal of Medicine* 385, no. 20 (November 11, 2021): 1868–80. https://doi.org/10.1056/NEJMoa2035790.

Oreskes, Naomi, and Erik Conway. *Merchants of Doubt: How a Handful of Scientists Obscured the Truth on Issues from Tobacco Smoke to Global Warming*. New York: Bloomsbury Press, 2010.

Panicola, Michael. "Does Hospital and Health System Consolidation Serve the Common Good?" *Journal of Moral Theology* 8, no. 1 (January 1, 2019): 63–75.

Panicola, Michael, and Rachelle Barina. "Catholic Health Care and Population Health: Insights from Catholic Social Thought." In *Catholic Bioethics and*

Social Justice, edited by M. Therese Lysaught and Michael McCarthy, 283–96. Collegeville, MN: Liturgical Press, 2018.

Panofsky, Aaron. *Misbehaving Science: Controversy and the Development of Behavior Genetics*. Chicago: University of Chicago Press, 2014.

Paul, Diane B. *The Politics of Heredity: Essays on Eugenics, Biomedicine, and the Nature-Nurture Debate*. Albany: SUNY Press, 1998.

Paul VI. *Octogesima Adveniens*. May 14, 1971. www.vatican.va/content/paul vi/en/apost_letters/documents/hf_p-vi_apl_19710514_octogesima adveniens.html.

Pavuk, Alexander. *Respectably Catholic and Scientific: Evolution and Birth Control between the World Wars*. Washington, DC: Catholic University of America Press, 2021.

Pearson, Karl. *The Grammar of Science*. London: A. and C. Black, 1911.

Pellegrino, Edmund D., and David C. Thomasma. *The Christian Virtues in Medical Practice*. Washington, DC: Georgetown University Press, 1996.

———. *For the Patient's Good: The Restoration of Beneficence in Health Care*. New York: Oxford University Press, 1988.

———. *A Philosophical Basis of Medical Practice: Toward a Philosophy and Ethic of the Healing Professions*. New York: Oxford University Press, 1982.

———. *The Virtues in Medical Practice*. New York: Oxford University Press, 1993.

Perrow, Charles. *Normal Accidents*. Princeton, NJ: Princeton University Press, 1999.

Pfeiffer, James, and Rachel Chapman. "An Anthropology of Aid in Africa." *The Lancet* 385, no. 9983 (May 30, 2015): 2144–45. https://doi.org/10.1016/S0140-6736(15)61013-3.

Plato. *Euthydemus*. Translated by Rosamund Sprague. In *Complete Works*, edited by John Cooper, 708–45. Indianapolis, IN: Hackett, 1997.

———. *Laws*. Translated by D. S. Hutchinson. In *Complete Works*, edited by John Cooper, 1318–1616. Indianapolis, IN: Hackett, 1997.

———. *Republic*. Translated by D. S. Hutchinson. In *Complete Works*, edited by John Cooper, 971–1223. Indianapolis, IN: Hackett, 1997.

Plomin, Robert. *Blueprint: How DNA Makes Us Who We Are*. Cambridge, MA: MIT Press, 2018.

Polanyi, Michael. *Personal Knowledge: Towards a Post-critical Philosophy*. Chicago: University of Chicago Press, 1962.

Pollan, Michael. *The Omnivore's Dilemma: A Natural History of Four Meals*. New York: Penguin, 2007.

Pontius the Deacon. "Life and Passion of Cyprian." Translated by Robert Ernest Wallis. In *Fathers of the Third Century: Hippolytus, Cyprian, Caius, Novatian, Appendix*, vol. 5 of *Ante-Nicene Fathers*, edited by Alexander Roberts and James Donaldson, 267–74. Peabody, MA: Hendrickson, 1994.

Pope, Stephen J. "Integral Human Development: From Paternalism to Accompaniment." *Theological Studies* 80, no. 1 (2019): 123–47.
Popejoy, Alice B., and Stephanie M. Fullerton. "Genomics Is Failing on Diversity." *Nature* 538, no. 7624 (October 2016): 161–64. https://doi.org/10.1038/538161a.
Popenoe, Paul. "Feeblemindedness." *Journal of Heredity* 6 (1915): 32–36.
Porter, Theodore. *Genetics in the Madhouse: The Unknown History of Human Heredity*. Princeton, NJ: Princeton University Press, 2020.
———. *Karl Pearson: The Scientific Life in a Statistical Age*. Princeton, NJ: Princeton University Press, 2006.
———. *The Rise of Statistical Thinking, 1820–1900*. Princeton, NJ: Princeton University Press, 1986.
Potter, Van Rensselaer. *Bioethics: Bridge to the Future*. Englewood Cliffs, NJ: Prentice-Hall, 1971.
Prainsack, Barbara. *Personalized Medicine: Empowered Patients in the 21st Century?* New York: New York University Press, 2018.
Prainsack, Barbara, and Alena Buyx. *Solidarity in Biomedicine and Beyond*. Cambridge: Cambridge University Press, 2017.
Prasad, Vinay. *Malignant: How Bad Policy and Bad Evidence Harm People with Cancer*. Baltimore: Johns Hopkins University Press, 2020.
President's Council on Bioethics [U.S.]. *Beyond Therapy: Biotechnology and the Pursuit of Happiness*. Washington, DC: President's Council on Bioethics, 2003.
"Prevent, v." In *OED Online*. Oxford University Press. www.oed.com/view/Entry/151073.
Price, Nathan D., Andrew T. Magis, John C. Earls, Gustavo Glusman, Roie Levy, Christopher Lausted, Daniel T. McDonald, et al. "A Wellness Study of 108 Individuals Using Personal, Dense, Dynamic Data Clouds." *Nature Biotechnology* 35, no. 8 (August 2017): 747–56. https://doi.org/10.1038/nbt.3870.
Price, W. Nicholson, II, Sara Gerke, and I. Glenn Cohen. "Potential Liability for Physicians Using Artificial Intelligence." *JAMA* 322, no. 18 (November 12, 2019): 1765–66. https://doi.org/10.1001/jama.2019.15064.
Proctor, Robert. *Golden Holocaust*. Berkeley: University of California Press, 2012.
———. *Racial Hygiene: Medicine under the Nazis*. Cambridge, MA: Harvard University Press, 1988.
Proctor, Robert, and Londa L. Schiebinger. *Agnotology: The Making and Unmaking of Ignorance*. Stanford, CA: Stanford University Press, 2008.
Provine, William. *The Origins of Theoretical Population Genetics*. Chicago: University of Chicago Press, 1971.
Public Discourse editors. "Moral Guidance on Prioritizing Care during a Pandemic." Joint Statement. *Public Discourse*, April 5, 2020. www.thepublicdiscourse.com/2020/04/62001/.

Public Health Agency of Sweden. "COVID-19 Recommendations," September 7, 2023. www.folkhalsomyndigheten.se/the-public-health-agency-of-sweden/communicable-disease-control/covid-19/how-to-protect-yourself-and-others-covid-19-recommendations/.

Rabinow, Paul. "Artificiality and Enlightenment: From Sociobiology to Biosociality." In *Essays on the Anthropology of Reason*, 91–111. Princeton, NJ: Princeton University Press, 1996.

———. *French DNA: Trouble in Purgatory*. Chicago: University of Chicago Press, 1999.

Ramsey, Paul. *Fabricated Man: The Ethics of Genetic Control*. New Haven, CT: Yale University Press, 1970.

———. *The Patient as Person: Explorations in Medical Ethics*. New Haven, CT: Yale University Press, 1970.

Reardon, Jenny. *The Postgenomic Condition*. Chicago: University of Chicago Press, 2017.

Rebillard, Eric. *In hora mortis: Évolution de la pastorale chrétienne de la mort aux IVe et Ve siècles dans l'Occident latin*. Bibliothèque des Ecoles Françaises d'Athènes et de Rome, fasc. 283. Rome: Ecole française de Rome, 1994.

Redberg, Rita F., and Mitchell H. Katz. "Statins for Primary Prevention: The Debate Is Intense, but the Data Are Weak." *JAMA Internal Medicine* 177, no. 1 (January 1, 2017): 21–23. https://doi.org/10.1001/jamainternmed.2016.7585.

Redfield, Peter. "Fluid Technologies: The Bush Pump, the LifeStraw® and Microworlds of Humanitarian Design." *Social Studies of Science* 46, no. 2 (April 2016): 159–83. https://doi.org/10.1177/0306312715620061.

Regalado, Antonio. "The World's First Gattaca Baby Tests Are Finally Here." *MIT Technology Review*, November 8, 2019.

Roberts, Dorothy. *Fatal Invention*. New York: New Press, 2011.

Romero, Miguel J. "Disability, Catholic Questions, and the Quandaries of Biomedicine and Secular Society." *National Catholic Bioethics Quarterly* 20, no. 2 (October 21, 2020): 277–310.

Rose, Geoffrey. *The Strategy of Preventive Medicine*. Oxford: Oxford University Press, 1992.

Rothman, David. *Strangers at the Bedside*. New York: Basic Books, 1991.

Rozier, Michael. "Collective Action on Determinants of Health: A Catholic Contribution." *Health Progress* 100, no. 5 (2019): 5–8.

———. "Global Public Health and Catholic Insights: Collaboration on Enduring Challenges." *Journal of Moral Theology* 1, CTEWC Book Series no. 1 (2021): 63–74.

———. "Religion and Public Health: Moral Tradition as Both Problem and Solution." *Journal of Religion and Health* 56 (2017): 1052–63.

———. "When Populations Become the Patient." *Health Progress* 98, no. 1 (February 2017): 5–8.
Russell, Louise. "Prevention vs. Cure: An Economist's Perspective on the Right Balance." In *Prevention vs. Treatment: What's the Right Balance?*, edited by Halley Faust and Paul Menzel, 56–76. New York: Oxford University Press, 2012.
Sachs, Jeffrey. *The End of Poverty: Economic Possibilities for Our Time*. New York: Penguin Books, 2006.
Sahlins, Marshall. *The Use and Abuse of Biology*. Ann Arbor: University of Michigan Press, 1976.
Sarosi, George. "The Tyranny of Guidelines." *Annals of Internal Medicine* 163 (2015): 562–63.
Savulescu, Julian. "Procreative Beneficence: Why We Should Select the Best Children." *Bioethics* 15, nos. 5/6 (2001): 413–26.
Sawyers, Charles L. "Herceptin: A First Assault on Oncogenes That Launched a Revolution." *Cell* 179, no. 1 (September 2019): 8–12. https://doi.org/10.1016/j.cell.2019.08.027.
Schelling, Thomas. "The Life You Save May Be Your Own." In *Problems in Public Expenditure Analysis*, edited by Samuel Chase, 127–61. Washington, DC: Brookings Institution, 1968.
Scherz, China. "Enduring the Awkward Embrace: Ontology and Ethical Work in a Ugandan Convent." *American Anthropologist* 120, no. 1 (2018): 102–12. https://doi.org/10.1111/aman.12968.
———. *Having People, Having Heart*. Chicago: University of Chicago Press, 2014.
———. "Let Us Make God Our Banker: Ethics, Temporality, and Agency in a Ugandan Charity Home." *American Ethnologist* 40, no. 4 (2013): 624–36.
Scherz, Paul. "Are Immortalized Cell Lines Artifacts? Commodification of Human Tissue and the COVID-19 Vaccine Debate." *National Catholic Bioethics Quarterly* 21, no. 2 (September 9, 2021): 219–30. https://doi.org/10.5840/ncbq202121223.
———. "Data Ethics, AI, and Accompaniment: The Dangers of Depersonalization in Catholic Health Care." *Theological Studies* 83, no. 2 (June 1, 2022): 271–92. https://doi.org/10.1177/00405639221096770.
———. "The Displacement of Human Judgment in Science: The Problems of Biomedical Research in an Age of Big Data." *Social Research* 86, no. 4 (2019): 957–76.
———. "Grief, Death, and Longing in Stoic and Christian Ethics." *Journal of Religious Ethics* 45, no. 1 (2017).
———. "Life as an Intelligence Test: Intelligence, Education, and Behavioral Genetics." *Culture, Medicine, and Psychiatry* 46, no. 1 (March 1, 2022): 59–75. https://doi.org/10.1007/s11013-021-09747-0.

———. "Living Indefinitely and Living Fully: Laudato Si' and the Value of the Present in Christian, Stoic, and Transhumanist Temporalities." *Theological Studies* 79, no. 2 (June 1, 2018): 356–75.

———. "The Mechanism and Applications of CRISPR-Cas9." *National Catholic Bioethics Quarterly* 17, no. 1 (June 7, 2017): 29–36. https://doi.org/10.5840/ncbq20171713.

———. "No Acceptable Losses: Risk, Prevention, and Justice." *Christian Bioethics* 29, no. 2 (August 1, 2023): 164–75. https://doi.org/10.1093/cb/cbad013.

———. "Risk, Health and Physical Enhancement: The Dangers of Health Care as Risk Reduction for Christian Bioethics." *Christian Bioethics* 26, no. 2 (2020): 145–62.

———. *Science and Christian Ethics.* Cambridge: Cambridge University Press, 2019.

———. *Tomorrow's Troubles: Risk, Anxiety, and Prudence in an Age of Algorithmic Governance.* Washington, DC: Georgetown University Press, 2022.

Schmitt, Carl. *Political Theology: Four Chapters on the Concept of Sovereignty.* Translated by George Schwab. Chicago: University of Chicago Press, 2006.

Schull, Natasha Dow. "The Data-Based Self: Self-Quantification and the Data-Driven (Good) Life." *Social Research* 86, no. 4 (2019): 909–30.

———. "Data for Life: Wearable Technology and the Design of Self-Care." *Biosocieties* 11, no. 3 (2016): 317–33.

Schwarze, Katharina, James Buchanan, Jilles M. Fermont, Helene Dreau, Mark W. Tilley, John M. Taylor, Pavlos Antoniou, et al. "The Complete Costs of Genome Sequencing: A Microcosting Study in Cancer and Rare Diseases from a Single Center in the United Kingdom." *Genetics in Medicine* 22, no. 1 (January 2020): 85–94. https://doi.org/10.1038/s41436-019-0618-7.

Scott, James C. *Seeing Like a State: How Certain Schemes to Improve the Human Condition Have Failed.* New Haven, CT: Yale University Press, 1999.

Scrinis, Gyorgy. "On the Ideology of Nutritionism." *Gastronomica* 8, no. 1 (2008): 39–48. https://doi.org/10.1525/gfc.2008.8.1.39.

Servick, Kelly. "Alzheimer's Drug Approved Despite Doubts about Effectiveness." *Science*, June 7, 2021. www.science.org/content/article/alzheimer-s-drug-approved-despite-doubts-about-effectiveness.

Shin, Sonya, Jennifer Furin, Jaime Bayona, Kedar Mate, Jim Yong Kim, and Paul Farmer. "Community-Based Treatment of Multidrug-Resistant Tuberculosis in Lima, Peru: 7 Years of Experience." *Social Science and Medicine* 59, no. 7 (October 2004): 1529–39. https://doi.org/10.1016/j.socscimed.2004.01.027.

Shrader-Frechette, Kristin. *Science Policy, Ethics, and Economic Methodology: Some Problems of Technology Assessment and Environmental-Impact Analysis.* Boston: Springer, 2013.

Singer, Peter. *The Life You Can Save: How to Do Your Part to End World Poverty*. New York: Random House, 2010.
Skloot, Rebecca. *The Immortal Life of Henrietta Lacks*. New York: Crown, 2010.
Slote, Michael. "Why Not Empathy?" In *Identified versus Statistical Lives: An Interdisciplinary Perspective*, edited by I. Glenn Cohen, Norman Daniels, and Nir M. Eyal, 150–60. Oxford: Oxford University Press, 2015.
Smalheiser, Neil R. "Informatics and Hypothesis-Driven Research." *EMBO Reports* 3, no. 8 (August 15, 2002): 702. https://doi.org/10.1093/embo-reports/kvf164.
Smith, James M. *Ireland's Magdalen Laundries and the Nation's Architecture of Containment*. Notre Dame, IN: University of Notre Dame Press, 2007.
Smith, Janet. "The Fake Theology behind Vaccine Mandates." *Crisis Magazine*, September 27, 2021. www.crisismagazine.com/2021/the-fake-theology-behind-vaccine-mandates.
Spencer, Hamish, and Diane B. Paul. "The Failure of a Scientific Critique: David Heron, Karl Pearson and Mendelian Eugenics." *British Journal for the History of Science* 31, no. 4 (1998): 441–52.
Stahl, Devan. *Disability's Challenge to Theology: Genes, Eugenics, and the Metaphysics of Modern Medicine*. Notre Dame, IN: University of Notre Dame Press, 2022.
Starr, Paul. *The Social Transformation of American Medicine: The Rise of a Sovereign Profession and the Making of a Vast Industry*. New York: Basic Books, 1984.
Stegenga, Jacob. *Medical Nihilism*. Oxford: Oxford University Press, 2018.
Stern, Alexandra. *Telling Genes: The Story of Genetic Counseling in America*. Baltimore: Johns Hopkins University Press, 2012.
Stevens, Hallam. *Life Out of Sequence*. Chicago: University of Chicago Press, 2013.
Stjernø, Steinar. *Solidarity in Europe: The History of an Idea*. Cambridge: Cambridge University Press, 2009.
Sullivan, Ezra. *Habits and Holiness: Ethics, Theology, and Biopsychology*. Washington, DC: Catholic University of America Press, 2021.
Sullivan, Richard, Olusegun Isaac Alatise, Benjamin O. Anderson, Riccardo Audisio, Philippe Autier, Ajay Aggarwal, Charles Balch, et al. "Global Cancer Surgery: Delivering Safe, Affordable, and Timely Cancer Surgery." *Lancet Oncology* 16, no. 11 (September 1, 2015): 1193–1224. https://doi.org/10.1016/S1470-2045(15)00223-5.
Sunstein, Cass. *Laws of Fear: Beyond the Precautionary Principle*. Cambridge: Cambridge University Press, 2005.
Sussman, Robert. *The Myth of Race*. Cambridge, MA: Harvard University Press, 2014.
Svenaeus, Fredrik. *The Hermeneutics of Medicine and the Phenomenology of Health: Steps towards a Philosophy of Medical Practice*. Dordrecht: Kluwer, 2000.

Sweet, Victoria. *God's Hotel: A Doctor, a Hospital, and a Pilgrimage to the Heart of Medicine.* New York: Riverhead Books, 2013.

Swensen, Stephen J., Gregg S. Meyer, Eugene C. Nelson, Gordon C. Hunt, David B. Pryor, Jed I. Weissberg, Gary S. Kaplan, et al. "Cottage Industry to Postindustrial Care: The Revolution in Health Care Delivery." *New England Journal of Medicine* 362, no. 5 (February 4, 2010): e12. https://doi.org/10.1056/NEJMp0911199.

Szakolczai, Árpád. *Max Weber and Michel Foucault: Parallel Life-Works.* New York: Routledge, 1998.

Taouk, Yamna, Matthew J. Spittal, Allison J. Milner, and Anthony D. LaMontagne. "All-Cause Mortality and the Time-Varying Effects of Psychosocial Work Stressors: A Retrospective Cohort Study Using the HILDA Survey." *Social Science and Medicine* 266 (December 2020): 113452. https://doi.org/10.1016/j.socscimed.2020.113452.

Taylor, Charles. *A Secular Age.* Cambridge, MA: Belknap Press, 2007.

Taylor, Lauren A. "How Do We Fund Flourishing? Maybe Not through Health Care." *Hastings Center Report* 48, no. S3 (2018): S62–66. https://doi.org/10.1002/hast.916.

Temkin, Owsei. *Galenism: The Rise and Decline of a Medical Philosophy.* Ithaca, NY: Cornell University Press, 1973.

Teslow, Tracy. *Constructing Race.* New York: Cambridge University Press, 2014.

Thaler, Richard, and Cass Sunstein. *Nudge: Improving Decisions about Health, Wealth, and Happiness.* New York: Penguin, 2009.

Thomas-Henkel, Caitlin, Allison Hamblin, and Taylor Hendricks. "Supporting a Culture of Health for High-Need, High-Cost Populations: Opportunities to Improve Models of Care for People with Complex Needs." Robert Wood Johnson Foundation and Center for Health Care Strategies, 2015. www.chcs.org/media/HNHC_CHCS_Report_Final-updated.pdf.

Thompson, Paul D., Gregory Panza, Amanda Zaleski, and Beth Taylor. "Statin-Associated Side Effects." *Journal of the American College of Cardiology* 67, no. 20 (May 24, 2016): 2395–2410. https://doi.org/10.1016/j.jacc.2016.02.071.

Titmuss, Richard Morris. *The Gift Relationship: From Human Blood to Social Policy.* New York: Pantheon Books, 1971.

Tollefson, Jeff. "These Experiments Could Lift Millions Out of Dire Poverty." *Nature* 606, no. 7915 (June 22, 2022): 640–42. https://doi.org/10.1038/d41586-022-01679-y.

Tonnies, Ferdinand. *Community and Civil Society.* Cambridge: Cambridge University Press, 2001.

Toombs, S. Kay. *The Meaning of Illness: A Phenomenological Account of the Different Perspectives of Physician and Patient.* Philosophy and Medicine. Dordrecht: Springer Netherlands, 1992. www.springer.com/gp/book/9780792315704.

Topol, Eric. *Deep Medicine: How Artificial Intelligence Can Make Healthcare Human Again*. New York: Basic Books, 2019.

Townes, Emilie M. *Breaking the Fine Rain of Death: African American Health Issues and a Womanist Ethic of Care*. Eugene, OR: Wipf and Stock, 2006.

U.K. Biobank. "Repeat Assessment: Participant Characteristics of Responders vs. Non-responders." Version 1.1. July 2014. https://biobank.ndph.ox.ac.uk/~bbdatan/repeat_assessment_characteristics_v1.pdf.

U.S. Preventive Services Task Force. "Final Recommendation Statement: Prostate Cancer: Screening," 2018. www.uspreventiveservicestaskforce.org/Page/Document/RecommendationStatementFinal/prostate-cancer-screening1.

———. "Statin Use for the Primary Prevention of Cardiovascular Disease in Adults: US Preventive Services Task Force Recommendation Statement." *JAMA* 328, no. 8 (August 23, 2022): 746–53. https://doi.org/10.1001/jama.2022.13044.

Verweij, Marcel. "How (Not) to Argue for the Rule of Rescue: Claims of Individuals versus Group Solidarity." In *Identified versus Statistical Lives: An Interdisciplinary Perspective*, edited by I. Glenn Cohen, Norman Daniels, and Nir M. Eyal, 150–60. Oxford: Oxford University Press, 2015.

Wade, Nicholas. *A Troublesome Inheritance*. New York: Penguin, 2014.

Walker, Joseph. "FDA Approves Bluebird's $2.8 Million Gene Therapy for Rare Blood Disease." *Wall Street Journal*, August 17, 2022. www.wsj.com/articles/fda-approves-bluebirds-2-8-million-gene-therapy-for-rare-blood-disease-11660759942.

Waters, Brent. *This Mortal Flesh: Incarnation and Bioethics*. Grand Rapids, MI: Brazos, 2009.

Weinberg, Alvin M. "Science and Trans-science." *Minerva* 10, no. 2 (April 1, 1972): 209–22. https://doi.org/10.1007/BF01682418.

Welch, H. Gilbert, Lisa Schwartz, and Steven Woloshin. *Overdiagnosed*. Boston: Beacon Press, 2011.

Witt, John. *The Accidental Republic*. Cambridge, MA: Harvard University Press, 2006.

Wolf, Gary. "Futurist Ray Kurzweil Pulls Out All the Stops (and Pills) to Live to Witness the Singularity." *WIRED* magazine, March 24, 2008. www.wired.com/2008/03/ff-kurzweil/.

World Health Organization. "Constitution of the World Health Organization." www.who.int/about/governance/constitution.

Wright, Addison V., James K. Nuñez, and Jennifer A. Doudna. "Biology and Applications of CRISPR Systems: Harnessing Nature's Toolbox for Genome Engineering." *Cell* 164, no. 1 (January 14, 2016): 29–44. https://doi.org/10.1016/j.cell.2015.12.035.

Yearley, Lee H. *Mencius and Aquinas: Theories of Virtue and Conceptions of Courage*. Albany: State University of New York Press, 1990.

Zigon, Jarrett. "Can Machines Be Ethical? On the Necessity of Relational Ethics and Empathic Attunement for Data-Centric Technologies." *Social Research* 86, no. 4 (2019): 1001–22.

Zubizarreta, E. H., E. Fidarova, B. Healy, and E. Rosenblatt. "Need for Radiotherapy in Low and Middle Income Countries: The Silent Crisis Continues." *Clinical Oncology* 27, no. 2 (February 1, 2015): 107–14. https://doi.org/10.1016/j.clon.2014.10.006.

Zuboff, Shoshana. *The Age of Surveillance Capitalism*. New York: PublicAffairs, 2019.

INDEX

A
Affordable Care Act, 63, 64, 67
Agamben, Giorgio, 147n26, 149n12, 152n8, 155n29, 158n29
algorithms, 33, 39
All of Us program, vii, 4, 34, 40
Anscombe, Elizabeth, 151n30
anxiety, viii, x, 8, 19–20, 80, 88–89, 93, 108, 110, 137n39
Aquinas, Thomas, 79, 111–12
Aristotle, 5, 56–57, 74, 90
artificial intelligence (AI), 70–72, 93, 121–22
artificial nutrition and hydration (ANH), 149n12, 150n28
asceticism, 11, 112–13
asylums, 26, 128–29
Austriaco, Nicanor, 78
autonomy, 45, 48–49, 67

B
bare life, 93–94, 149n12
Berwick, Donald, 66, 72
BiDil (drug), 37
bioethics, 41–52
biopolitics, 145n13 (chap. 6), 153n16
biopower, 145n13 (chap. 6), 147n26
blood pressure, viii, 15, 16, 20
Body Mass Index (BMI), 8

Bourdieu, Pierre, 109
Braswell, Harold, 130–31

C
cancer
  breast, 9, 17–18, 43
  and genetics, 32–33
  moonshot vs. groundshot, 122–23
  prostate, 19–22
  screening, 17–18, 19–20, 65, 77
  and tumor sequencing, 117–20
Canguilhem, Georges, 134n18
cardiovascular disease, 9, 14–17, 21, 24
Cassel, Eric, 50
Cassian, John, 112
Catholic casuistry of ordinary and extraordinary means, 75–80
charity, 88, 89, 111, 130, 131, 132
cholesterol, 15, 78
Clement of Alexandria, 111
clinical encounter/ethos, 7, 13–14, 46–47, 135n21
Collins, Francis, vii
colonoscopy, 21
common good, 60, 74, 78, 81, 90, 110, 144n8
Congregation for the Doctrine of the Faith, 77
cost-effectiveness, 61, 64–65, 83, 84

191

courage, 88, 110, 132
Covid-19 pandemic, xi, 61, 89, 94
   vaccine, 78–80
cybernetics, 30, 33
Cyprian of Carthage, 87–89

D
DALYs, 61
Darwin, Charles, 26
Davis, Joseph, 101
deskilling, 71–72
diagnostic odyssey, 115–16
diathesis, 27, 30
diet, 107–9
disability, 6, 134n19

E
Ehrenreich, Barbara, 81
electronic medical records (EMR), 67, 68, 70
eugenics, 26–27, 29, 31, 59–60, 84–85, 152n11
Ewald, Francois, 154n13

F
faith, 87–89
Farmer, Paul, 92–93, 151n3
fasting, 112–13
Foucault, Michel, 145n13 (chap. 6), 147n26, 152n8, 153n16, 158n29, 158n31
Framingham Heart Study, 15–16, 33
Francis, Pope, 88, 136n36, 137n38, 152n7, 153n10

G
Galen, 106, 110
Galton, Francis, 27, 35
genetics, 4
   determinism, 30, 32, 33, 35
   disease, congenital, 115–17
   Mendelian, 28–29
   molecular, 29–31
   population, 29, 32
   screening and testing, 24, 31, 81, 85
   therapy, 31, 114, 116
   whole-genome sequencing, 115, 142n38
Gnosticism, 10–12, 112, 113, 136n36
Gould, Stephen Jay, 44
greed, 56–57
guidelines, medical, 56, 71

H
habits, 106
health, 133n3 (chap. 1)
   as absence of disease, 4–7
   as absence of risk, 7–12, 55
   obligation to preserve, 74–82
   political concern with, 59–62, 100, 102–3
   as a subordinate good, 112
   World Health Organization definition, 55–56, 60
Health Maintenance Organizations (HMO), 65, 66
heart disease. *See* cardiovascular disease
Herceptin, 118
high-risk patients and their programs, 83, 120–22, 129, 130
HIV, 83, 92–93
hospice, 128, 130–31
hospitals, 126
Human Genome Project, vii, 31–32, 35
Human Longevity Incorporated, 58
humors, 106
hypertension. *See* blood pressure

I
identified lives, 91–92
Illich, Ivan, 134n15, 156n10, 160n8
insurance, 64, 84, 104, 139n4, 146n17, 152n9

J
Judaism, and obligation to maintain health, 77
justice, 47, 51–52

K
Knight, Frank, 42–43
Kurzweil, Ray, 109–10

L
Laguna Honda Hospital, 126–28, 129, 130
Leo, Pope, 113
loneliness, 101

M
mammograms, viii, 8, 18, 21, 41, 67
McKenny, Gerald, 136n33
McKeown, Thomas, 85
medicalization, 52, 59, 101–5
memento mori, 110
Mercy House, 124–25, 128, 130
metrics, 66, 67, 69, 70, 72, 121–22, 125
Mol, Annemarie, 67–68

N
National Institute for Health and Care Excellence (NICE), 65
nongovernmental organizations (NGOs), 104
number needed to treat (NNT), 22–23, 82, 120
nutrition research, 108

O
obesity and food policy, 103, 109
100,000 Genomes Project, 115–16
orphanages, 128–29

P
pain, 5, 6, 76
Pap smears, 18
paternalism, 47, 48–49
patient advocacy groups, 57
Paul, 10–11, 136n33
Pearson, Karl, 27, 28, 30, 34, 35
Pellegrino, Edmund, 133n2 (chap. 1), 135n21, 155n22
perfect duties, 76, 79
persistent vegetative state (PVS), 149n12
pharmaceutical industry, 16–17
Pioneer 100 Wellness Project, 3–4, 58
Plato, 81, 108–9, 110
pollution, 60
Polygenic Risk Score (PRS), 34, 41–42, 43–44, 85, 121
polypharmacy, 58, 72
population, viii, x, 16, 21–23, 25–27, 34, 35–36, 38, 42–44, 49, 50, 52, 69, 85–86, 89, 152n8
population health programs, 83
preferential option for the poor, 151n3
pregnancy, 135n30
pride, 112, 113
procreative beneficence, 85
prudence, ix–xi, 9, 68–72, 80, 121–22, 132
PSA test, 8, 19–20

Q
QALYs, 61
Quantified Self (QS), 9, 110
Quetelet, Adolphe, 26

R
race, 26, 37–38, 40–42, 135n24
rationing, 64–65
reductionism, 30, 33, 35–36, 47, 49–51
regimen, 106–13
resurrection, 136n35
risk factors, 15–16, 34, 100

Rose, Geoffrey, 99, 120
Rozier, Michael, 45–46, 49, 156n15

S
Sanchez, Tomas, 77
Sarosi, George, 69–70
scalability, 130–31
Scherz, China, 124–25
shared decision-making, 68
side effects, 19–21, 56, 58, 61, 99, 119
single nucleotide polymorphism (SNP), 34, 41
slow medicine, 127, 130
social determinants of health, 50–52, 59, 99–105
solidarity, 89–90, 92, 113, 116–17
statins, 20–22, 77, 120
statistical lives, 91–92
statistical other, 89
statistics, 8, 9, 15–16, 22, 25–29, 37–38, 42–44, 152n8
Svenaeus, Fredrik, 5
Sweet, Victoria, 126–27, 129, 130

T
Taft, William Howard, 60
Taylor, Charles, 160n8
temperance, ix, 11, 111–12, 132
Titmuss, Richard, 154n13
Tonnies, Ferdinand, 155n24
transhumanism, 11, 134n17

V
value-based care, 66–67, 69, 70, 72
variants of unknown significance (VUS), 116
Venter, Craig, 58
virtue, ix–x, 7, 46, 81, 90, 109, 130–31, 132, 134n6, 151n30
Vitoria, Francisco de, 76

W
wellness program, 63, 72–73, 80, 130

Y
yearly checkup, 13, 21

PAUL SCHERZ

is the Our Lady of Guadalupe Professor of Theology
at the University of Notre Dame.
He is the author and editor of several books, including
*The Evening of Life: The Challenges of Aging and
Dying Well* (University of Notre Dame Press, 2020).